The AAMT Book of Style
for Medical Transcription
Second Edition

Editor Peg Hughes, CMT

Contributing Authors Linda A. Byrne, CMT
Diane S. Heath, CMT
Brenda J. Hurley, CMT
Kathy Rockel, CMT
Claudia Tessier, CAE, CMT

AMERICAN ASSOCIATION FOR MEDICAL TRANSCRIPTION

The AAMT Book of Style for Medical Transcription

ISBN 0-935229-38-8

Author of the original *AAMT Book of Style for Medical Transcription*
Claudia Tessier, CAE, CMT

Design and Layout
John Campbell

Index
Mara Pinckard, Canyon View Indexing

American Association for Medical Transcription
A Nonprofit Professional Corporation
100 Sycamore Avenue
Modesto, CA 95354-0550
Phone: 209-527-9620
Fax: 209-527-9633
Email: aamt@aamt.org
Web: www.aamt.org

Printed in the United States of America
Last digit indicates print number: 10   9   8   7   6   5   4   3   2

To all medical transcriptionists,
most especially to those who place
quality before quantity and who practice
medical transcription as both an art and a science.

Table of Contents

Acknowledgements

Countless medical transcriptionists have played a role in the revision of *The AAMT Book of Style* in their pursuit of quality healthcare documentation. Whether by calling attention to a shortfall or by contacting the AAMT Help Desk for clarification of a style point, they have advocated for an improved style manual. We thank them all.

We are particularly indebted to the following individuals, who reviewed the entire draft manuscript and provided numerous helpful suggestions and comments.

Susan Bartolucci, CMT
Carrie Boatman, CMT
Aleena Campbell
Claudia Crickmore, CMT
Margie Kahn, CMT
Audrey Klocke Heintz, CMT
Ann Stanton, CMT

Special thanks go to John Dirckx, MD, not only for his invaluable assistance in reviewing the draft manuscript, but also for his appreciation of and involvement with medical transcriptionists for many years.

PH

Introduction

As the professional association for medical transcription, AAMT is the recognized leader in acknowledging and establishing medical transcription styles, forms, and practices. This book represents AAMT's most complete conclusions for a wide variety of such topics. We reach our conclusions through research and experience, through logic and common sense, and through the experience and expertise of a great many medical transcriptionists. MT supervisors, educators, and students have also had a hand in the creation of this book.

We urge you and other MT practitioners, students, teachers, supervisors, and originators of dictation to adopt our forms, styles, and practices, but we take the role of persuader, not enforcer. AAMT's conclusions are widely accepted because our reputation for quality and exactness has established AAMT as the recognized authority in the world of medical transcription. By incorporating our conclusions into your practices, you have our experience and reputation upon which to justify your decisions and our materials with which to document them.

Whether you adopt *The AAMT Book of Style* in its entirety or piecemeal, keep in mind that consistency of style choice in a given document—for example, spelling the abbreviation for the United States with or without periods—gives your work added credibility.

As physicians and other caregivers dictate reports, they are often reading abbreviated, handwritten notes, and the MT's job is to translate any shorthand-type dictation into a more formal narrative that becomes part of the medicolegal record. Hence, our approach is to avoid nonstandard abbreviations and to avoid the use of symbols pronounced as words (see the discussion of *greater than*, for an example). There is a constant tension between transcribing just what is dictated and employing a more standardized language and format in an effort to establish "best practices" in healthcare documentation.

New in the Second Edition

Ever since the publication of the first edition of *The AAMT Book of Style*, we have collected the comments and suggestions of our readers in order to make the second edition more complete and useful. One notable change is the recommendation to use numerals throughout medical reports rather than spelling out certain numbers. The frequency of calls and emails to our office on this topic demonstrated the confusion MTs face when deciding whether it should be a *six-day history of fever and chills* or a *6-day history of fever and chills*. The MT can facilitate clear and prompt communication about a patient by simply using a numeral.

Introduction

While the *Book of Style* focuses more on style than on the practice of medical transcription, there are many instances where styles become practices, and practices create styles. A case in point is the material from the Institute for Safe Medication Practices (Appendix B). By adopting their guidelines in this second edition, AAMT has changed its style recommendations for writing certain dosage instructions (using *daily* instead of *q.d.*, for example, even when the abbreviation is dictated).

The establishment of governmental regulations related to the Health Insurance Portability and Accountability Act of 1996 (HIPAA) has also forced us to look at practice in the area of confidentiality and security, and innovations in technology have brought a whole new meaning to the word *editing*.

The *Book of Style* is not a terminology book, although there is certainly a great deal of overlap between style and terminology. We have generally avoided giving definitions of terms and word lists; however, we have bent this rule from time to time. For example, in the second edition we have stated a preference for the spelling of *disk* over *disc*.

The request that we make the book more "user friendly" was often expressed by users of the first edition. Therefore, the printed version of the second edition of *The AAMT Book of Style* is wider, allowing it to lie flat when open. Its type style and format are easier on the eye, and it contains a complete index for quick referencing. In addition, we have repeated information in more than one location when doing so makes the information easier to find. We have also added useful hints in the margins—tips that will help you remember a key point. And for those users who have a special interest in jumping to their favorite topics, we have used icons in the margins that will help to quickly identify points of grammar, punctuation, and usage.

The Third Edition

Before the second edition is even on the shelf, we are already thinking ahead to the third edition, so please keep those questions and suggestions coming. Send your comments to

AAMT Book of Style
100 Sycamore Avenue
Modesto, CA 95354-0550
Fax 209-527-9633
Email aamt@aamt.org

Thank you for adding this publication to your library. Use it in good health!

Peg Hughes, CMT
Editor

A

a, an

The indefinite articles are *a* and *an*, and the definite article is *the*.

> *a* chair *(may be any chair)*
> *the* chair *(a specific, or definite, chair)*

See articles

before consonants, h's, u sounds, vowels

Use *a* before a consonant, a sounded (aspirate) *h*, or a long *u* sound. Use *an* before a vowel or an unsounded *h*.

> a patient
> a hemorrhoid
> a unit
> an indication
> an hour
> a 1-mile run
> a CMT
> an 8-hour delay
> an MT

HINT: Pronunciation determines whether a word is preceded by *a* or *an;* this is most useful with abbreviations and numerals.

abbreviations, acronyms, brief forms

Abbreviations, acronyms, and brief forms are often used in medical dictation to speed up communication, but they frequently create confusion instead. While the originator may think that dictating the abbreviation *AML* is the fastest way to communicate *acute myelocytic leukemia*, medical transcriptionists know better. They face the dilemma: Does *AML* mean acute monocytic leukemia, acute myeloblastic leukemia, acute myelocytic leukemia, acute myelogenous leukemia, acute myeloid leukemia, or perhaps even some less common alternative? In the numerous publications devoted to translating medical abbreviations, abbreviations with a single meaning appear to be in the minority.

Clarity of communication is essential. Avoid the use of abbreviations, acronyms, and brief forms except for internationally recognized and accepted units of measure and for widely recognized terms and symbols. Do not use any that readers will not immediately recognize. Unless the abbreviation, acronym, or brief form is so widely used that it has in essence become a term in its own right, use the expanded term first, followed by its abbreviated form in parentheses. Then use the abbreviated form throughout the remainder of the document.

Some abbreviations, particularly with respect to medication orders, have proven to be dangerous. For example, the *U* in *insulin 6 U* could possibly be misread as a zero, or a medication that is to be given once a day may mistakenly be given four times a day if *q.d.* were misread as *q.i.d.* These types of errors can and do happen and have at times caused fatalities.

Organizations involved in identifying and preventing such problems include the United States Pharmacopeia (USP), the Institute for Safe Medication Practices (ISMP), the US Food and Drug Administration (FDA), and the National Coordinating Council for Medication Error Reporting and Prevention (NCC MERP). ISMP has published a list of dangerous abbreviations and dose designations as reported to the USP-ISMP Medication Errors Reporting Program, and AAMT has chosen to promote the adoption of this list (***See*** Appendix B: Dangerous Abbreviations).

There is no nationally recognized list of approved abbreviations for use in medical reports, nor does AAMT propose such a list. However, it is important to note that the Joint Commission on Accreditation of Healthcare Organizations (JCAHO) requires that in order to be accredited a hospital should use uniform data definitions whenever possible; they note that an abbreviation list (which might be interpreted as a list of abbreviations to avoid) is one way to meet this requirement.

acronyms

Acronyms (and initialisms) are abbreviations formed from the initial letters of each of the successive words or major parts of a compound term or of selected letters of a word or phrase.

Acronyms are usually pronounced as words *(AIDS, GERD, LASIK)*, while initialisms are not *(ALS, CPK, HCV)*.

Some acronyms evolve into words in their own right.

laser   light amplification by stimulated emission of radiation (*initially written as* LASER)

When an acronym form of a term is dictated, either use the acronym or transcribe the term in full, as appropriate. Follow the guidelines for abbreviation usage.

brief forms

Shortened forms of words.

Transcribe brief forms as dictated if they are commonly used and widely recognized, but extend them in headings, diagnoses, and operative titles. Lowercase the brief form unless the extended form is routinely capitalized. Do not use an ending period. Form the plural by adding *s* (no apostrophe) to the term itself or to its accompanying noun if the term is an adjective.

phone   telephone
exam   examination
Pap smear Papanicolaou smear

abbreviating terms dictated in full

Do not use an abbreviation, acronym, or brief form when a term is dictated in full except for units of measure, e.g., milligrams, centimeters. Such abbreviations not only are universally known and accepted but are preferable because they communicate their meaning more quickly and succinctly than their extended forms. Use such abbreviations even in diagnostic statements or operative titles, for they are not themselves the diagnosis or operation name. *See* in diagnoses and operative titles *and* with numerals *below*.

> The patient reported a history of coronary artery bypass graft.
> (*not* CABG, *unless dictated* CABG *or* cabbage)

> D: The patient was prepared and draped.
> T: The patient was prepared and draped.
> *not* The patient was prepped and draped. (*unless dictated* prepped)

abbreviations with multiple or uncertain meanings

When an abbreviated diagnosis, conclusion, or operative title is dictated and the abbreviation used is not familiar or has multiple meanings, the meaning may be discerned if the originator uses the extended term elsewhere in the dictation or if the content of the report somehow makes the meaning obvious. If the extended form cannot be determined in this way and there is easy and immediate access to the patient's record or to the person who dictated the report, the MT should use these as resources to determine the meaning. If these attempts are unsuccessful, the abbreviated form should be transcribed as dictated, then flagged, requesting that the originator provide the extended form.

at the beginning of a sentence

A sentence may begin with a dictated abbreviation, acronym, or brief form (except units of measure), or such abbreviated forms may be extended.

> WBC was 9200.
> *or* White blood count was 9200.

> Exam was delayed.
> *or* Examination was delayed.

But never begin a sentence with a lowercase letter, such as *pH*.

in diagnoses and operative titles

Write out an abbreviation or acronym in full if it is used in the admission, discharge, preoperative, or postoperative diagnosis; consultative conclusion; or operative title. These are critical points of information, and their meanings must be clear to assure accurate communication for patient care, reimbursement, statistical purposes, and medicolegal documentation.

> D: Operation Performed: MID-CAB.
> T: Operation Performed: Minimally invasive direct coronary artery bypass.

Non-disease-entity abbreviations accompanying diagnostic and procedure statements may be used if dictated. (Note that it is preferable to abbreviate units of measure.)

> Operation: Removal of 3-cm nevus, lateral aspect, right knee.

If unable to translate an abbreviation or acronym that appears in a diagnosis or operative title, the MT should leave a blank and flag the report, asking the originator to translate it.

elsewhere in report

Within the narrative portion of the report, abbreviations, acronyms, and brief forms that are common and readily understood may be transcribed as dictated, or they may be written in full. Abbreviations and acronyms that are not easily recognized should be transcribed in full.

If unable to determine the abbreviation's meaning, the MT should transcribe it as dictated (or leave a blank) and then flag the report, asking the originator to translate it.

with numerals

Abbreviate units of measure, even if dictated in full, if they are accompanied by a numeral.

> 2.5 cm
>
> 3 g/dL

Where possible, avoid separating a numeral from its associated unit of measure or accompanying abbreviation; that is, keep the numeral and unit of measure together at line breaks.

> ....The specimen measured 4 cm in diameter.
>
> *or* ....The specimen measured 4 cm in diameter.
>
> *not* ....The specimen measured 4 cm in diameter

business and organization names

For acronyms and initialisms representing businesses and organizations, follow the style preference of the business or organization.

JCAHO　Joint Commission on Accreditation of
　　　　　Healthcare Organizations

APhA　　American Pharmaceutical Association

capitalization of acronyms

Capitalize all letters of most acronyms, but when they are extended, do not capitalize the words from which they are formed unless they are proper names.

AIDS　　(**a**cquired **immuno**de**f**iciency **s**yndrome)

BiPAP　　(**bi**lateral **p**ositive **a**irway **p**ressure)

TURP　　(**t**rans**u**rethral **r**esection of **p**rostate)

When acronyms become words in their own right, they sometimes evolve into lowercase form. Many users of these terms are not aware that such terms are acronyms and do not know what terms the letters represent.

laser　　(**l**ight **a**mplification by **s**timulated **e**mission of **r**adiation)

Check appropriate references (dictionaries, abbreviation books) to determine current preferred forms and usage.

periods

Do not use periods within or at the end of most abbreviations, including acronyms, abbreviated units of measure, and brief forms. Use a period at the end of abbreviated English units of measure if they may be misread without the period. Better still, write out most English units of measure, thereby avoiding this use of a period at the end of an abbreviation.

wbc

WBC

mg

exam

prep

inch *preferred to* in. (Do not use *in* meaning *inch* without a period.)

Do not use periods with abbreviated academic degrees and professional credentials.

BA	PA-C
CMT	PhD
MD	RN

However, use periods in lowercase drug-related abbreviations. (***See** section on* drug terminology *for a more complete list.*)

b.i.d.

q.4 h.

p.o.

p.r.n.

Periods may be used with courtesy titles (e.g., *Mr., Mrs.*) and following *Jr.* and *Sr.*, although there is a trend toward dropping them; either remains acceptable, but be consistent.

Occasionally, an entity will use periods in its own acronym; follow its preference.

> *A.D.A.M. Student Atlas of Anatomy*, published by Lippincott Williams & Wilkins

If a sentence terminates with an abbreviation that requires a period, do not add another period.

> He takes Valium 5 mg q.a.m.
> *not* He takes Valium 5 mg q.a.m..

plurals

Use a lowercase *s* without an apostrophe to form the plural of capitalized abbreviations, acronyms, and brief forms.

> EEGs
> PVCs
> CABGs
> exams

Use *'s* to form the plural of lowercase abbreviations.

> rbc's

Use *'s* to form the plural of single-letter abbreviations.

> X's

possession

Add *'s* to most abbreviations or acronyms to show possession.

> The AMA's address is...
> AAMT's position paper on full disclosure states...

productivity considerations

A decision on whether to use an abbreviation should be made on the basis of communication and usage, not for financial reasons. Abbreviations, acronyms, and brief forms should not be expanded simply for the purpose of increasing productivity count. Nor should words be abbreviated in an attempt to reduce the amount of text.

If an employer or client insists on the excessive use of abbreviations, the MT should retain some evidence of the directive.

unusual abbreviations

Some abbreviations do not follow the usual pattern of all capitals or the alternative of all lowercase letters. Learn the most common exceptions, and consult appropriate references for guidance.

> pH
> aVL
> PhD
> RPh

See drug terminology
   Appendix B: Dangerous Abbreviations

-able, -ible

There is no shortcut to determining the spelling of a term ending in *-able* or *-ible*. Consult appropriate references (i.e., dictionaries) for guidance.

abort, abortion, abortus

See obstetrics

a.c.

Abbreviation for *ante cibum* (before food), sometimes used in reference to drug administration.

See drug terminology

punctuation

accent marks

Also known as diacritics or diacritical marks, accent marks serve as a guide to pronunciation. They are usually omitted in medical transcription because of technology limitations, the likelihood of misuse, and the fact that they are not essential to communication.

Use of accents is required rarely, such as in proper names, but even then they should be omitted if technology does not permit their proper use.

When using accent marks, check appropriate references (dictionaries) to determine accurate usage. Examples of accent marks encountered in medical transcription include the following:

accent	*example*
acute	Calvé-Perthes disease
cedilla	François Chaussier sign
circumflex	bête rouge
dieresis	Laënnec
grave	boutonnière deformity
ring	Ångstrom
tilde	jalapeño
umlaut	Grüntzig catheter
virgule	Brønsted acid

Many words once spelled with accents no longer require them, e.g., resume, facade, cooperation, naive, fiancee.

Never enter accent marks by hand.

acting (as part of a title)

Capitalize when part of a capitalized title.

Charles Woodward, MD, who is acting chief of staff, ...

Today's speaker is Acting Chief of Staff Charles Woodward, MD.

Charles Woodward, MD
Acting Chief of Staff
Memorial Hospital
Main Street
Anytown, Any State, USA

addresses

See correspondence

adjectives

Adjectives modify nouns and sometimes pronouns.

Use commas to separate two or more adjectives if each modifies the noun alone. Do not place a comma between the last adjective and the modified noun.

Physical exam reveals a pleasant, cooperative, slender lady in no acute distress.
The abdomen is soft, nontender, and supple.

HINT: If you can replace the comma between adjectives with *and*, the comma is necessary.

However, do not place a comma after an adjective that modifies a combination of the adjective(s) and noun that follow it.

This 54-year-old Caucasian female was referred to my office for evaluation.
She did not have audible paroxysmal tachycardia.

Use commas to set off an adjective or adjectival phrase directly following the noun it modifies.

> Diagnosis: Fracture, left tibia.
>
> He has degenerative arthritis, left knee, with increasing inability to cope.
>
> Blood cultures, all of which were negative, were drawn at 4-hour intervals.

Some words can function as adjectives or adverbs, depending on how they are used.

adjective	*adverb*
hard work	play *hard*
light color	travel *light*

See compound modifiers

adnexa

Appendages or adjunct parts. The uterine adnexa consist of the ovaries, tubes, and ligaments. The optical adnexa are the lids, lashes, brows, conjunctival sacs, lacrimal apparatus, and extrinsic muscles.

Adnexa is always plural, even when referring to only one side.

> The adnexa are normal.
>
> Left adnexa are normal.
>
> The ocular adnexa are normal on the right.

adverbs

Adverbs modify verbs, adjectives, and other adverbs.

Some but not all adverbs end in *-ly*.

sterilely

Some words can function as adverbs or adjectives, depending on how they are used.

adverb	*adjective*
play *hard*	*hard* work
travel *light*	*light* color

An adverb may be placed between the parts of a compound verb, provided it does not obstruct the meaning.

He will routinely return for followup.

It is increasingly acceptable to split an infinitive verb (e.g., the verb *to be*) with an adverb. Transcribe as dictated, provided the phrasing does not obstruct the meaning.

The test was expected to definitively determine the diagnosis.

squinting modifiers

A squinting modifier is an adverb that is placed in such a way that it can be interpreted as modifying more than one word. If the intended meaning can be determined, recast the sentence so that the modifier clearly relates to the appropriate word. See how the placement of *only* in the following sentence changes the meaning.

He only walked 2 blocks. *(He only walked, not ran.)*
Only he walked 2 blocks. *(Only he, not anyone else, walked 2 blocks.)*
He walked only 2 blocks. *(He didn't walk more than 2 blocks.)*

So the squinting modifier *only* in "He only walked 2 blocks" should be moved so that the sentence reads "He walked only 2 blocks."

conjunctive adverbs
See conjunctions

affect, effect
These terms often sound alike when dictated, but their usage and meanings are not interchangeable. *Affect* is usually a verb, and *effect* is usually a noun. In medicine either of these terms may be a verb or noun, with a multitude of meanings, and their differences in usage and meaning should be learned.

affect
As a verb, *affect* (pronounced af-féct) means to influence or change.

She suffers from a neuropathy affecting her upper extremities.
The warm encouragement of the patient's wife positively affected his outcome.

As a noun, *affect* (pronounced áf-fect) means an expressed or observed emotion or feeling.

The patient displayed a flat affect.
Her affect did not change throughout the course of the interview.

effect

As a verb, *effect* means to bring about or cause to happen.

> We plan to effect a decrease in the size of the tumor using adjunctive therapy.
>
> The medication effected relief.

As a noun, *effect* means result.

> The effect of the treatment was pronounced.
>
> A mass effect was seen on x-ray.

African American

Both *African American* and *black* are acceptable designations for Americans of African heritage. Use the term dictated.

> The patient is a 35-year-old African American man.

See sociocultural designations

age referents

Use the term that is dictated unless it is a derogatory form or it is clearly wrong. However, in more formal writing, use the following guidelines.

neonates and newborns

Children from birth to 1 month of age. May also be referred to as boys and girls and children.

infants

Children from 1 month to 24 months (2 years) of age. May also be referred to as boys and girls and children.

child, children

Boys and girls aged 2 to 13 years. These terms may also be used for those from birth to 13 years. May also be referred to as boys and girls.

adolescents, youths, teenagers

Boys and girls aged 13 through 17 years. May also be referred to as boys and girls.

boys and girls

Neonates, children and adolescents, i.e., people from birth through 17 years. May also be referred to as neonates, newborns, children, adolescents, youths, and teenagers, depending on their age.

adults

People aged 18 years or older. May also be referred to as men and women.

man, men; woman, women

Adults, i.e., people aged 18 years or older. May also be referred to as adults.

ages

Use numerals to express ages, except at the beginning of a sentence.

37-year-old man
3½-year-old child
3-year 7-month-old girl

at the beginning of a sentence

Recast the sentence or write out the number.

D: 7-year-old patient who comes in today for...
T: A 7-year-old patient who comes in today for...
or This 7-year-old patient comes in today for...
or Seven-year-old patient who comes in today for...

as adjectival phrases

Use hyphens if the adjectival phrase precedes the noun.

> 15-year-old boy *not* 15 year old boy
> 13-year-olds *not* 13 year olds

Do not use hyphens when the phrase stands alone.

> The patient, who is 15 years old, ...
> *not* 15-years-old

Use a hyphen in a phrase in which the noun following the phrase is implied, or in a phrase that is serving as a noun. Alternatively, edit to a form that does not require hyphens.

> The patient, a 33-year-old, was pregnant for the fifth time.
> (*The word* patient *or* woman *is implied following* 33-year-old.)
> *or* The patient, 33 years old, was pregnant for the fifth time.

as decade references

Use numerals plus *s* to refer to decades. Do not use an apostrophe.

> The patient is in her 50s. (*not* 50's, *not* fifties)

a.k.a.

Abbreviation meaning *also known as*. Use lowercase letters with periods to distinguish from *AKA*, meaning above-knee amputation.

> The report was published by the National Academies, a.k.a. National Academy of Sciences, National Academy of Engineering, National Research Council, Institute of Medicine.

alfa

Variant spelling for *alpha*, used especially in generic drug names. Check references for applications.

alfa interferon

allergies

Some institutions use capitals or bold type to draw attention to a patient's allergies. Regular type is, of course, also acceptable. Do not underline or use italics; either reduces readability.

ALLERGIES: penicillin and aspirin.

or ALLERGIES: PENICILLIN AND ASPIRIN.

or **ALLERGIES: penicillin and aspirin.**

but not <u>ALLERGIES: penicillin and aspirin.</u>

and not *ALLERGIES: penicillin and aspirin.*

Note: ASTM's *E2184, Standard Specification for Healthcare Document Formats* calls for all major section headings in the report as well as allergies (the heading **and** the substance to which the individual is allergic) to be expressed in all capital letters. The standard does not specify bold type, with the understanding that technology does not always support special formatting.

ALLERGIES
PENICILLIN.

See formats

alphanumeric terms

Terms composed of letters and numerals; they may include symbols. Rules vary. Check appropriate topics within this text for guidance, or other references if the topic is not covered here.

> L4-5
> T4
> 3M

alternate, alternative

Soundalikes that are sometimes interchangeable but not always. Beware of misuse.

alternate

Alternate, meaning *occurring in turns,* can be either a verb or an adjective.

> She will alternate acetaminophen with naproxen to avoid GI symptoms.

In the following examples, *alternate* and *alternating* are used as adjectives.

> Daunorubicin will be administered on alternate Mondays.
> *(every other Monday)*

> Valium was given in alternating doses of 5 mg and 10 mg.

> Rapid alternating movements within normal limits.

alternative

Alternative, meaning *choice,* can be either a noun or an adjective.

> The alternatives were chemotherapy and radiation therapy.
> Alternative forms being considered include...

alternative forms

Styles and practices in medical transcription may vary widely. Some styles are acceptable but not necessarily preferred; others are not acceptable because they are not correct. This book attempts to present forms that are the most preferred, while acknowledging some alternative acceptable forms.

Some forms that are widely used and/or well documented are not correct. For example, *Verres* needle continues to be both widely used and documented, but the correct form is *Veress*. Thus, *Verres* is not an acceptable alternative form.

although, though

When used as conjunctions, *although* and *though* are considered interchangeable. However, when *though* is used an adverb it cannot be replaced by *although*.

although

A subordinating conjunction that joins a dependent clause to a main clause.

When the *although* clause precedes the main clause, it is usually followed by a comma. When it follows the main clause, it may be preceded by a comma if needed for clarity and understanding; the comma may be omitted if doing so does not confuse the reader. Note that in each of the following three examples, *though* can be used in place of *although*.

> Although he was frightened, the child cooperated fully with the exam.
> The child cooperated fully with the exam although he was frightened.
> *or* The child cooperated fully with the exam, although he was frightened.

though

An adverb, but widely used as a conjunction (equivalent to *although*). It is not necessary to set *though* off by commas unless there is a break in continuity or the need for a pause in reading.

> It was difficult for him. He did it though.
> Even though he was frightened, he did it.

a.m., AM; p.m., PM

Acceptable abbreviations for *ante meridiem* (before noon) and *post meridiem* (after noon), with the lowercase forms being preferred. Formal publications use small capitals, which, if available, may also be used in transcription.

> 8:15 a.m. *or* 8:15 AM *or* 8:15 A.M.

Do not use these abbreviations with a phrase such as *in the morning, in the evening, tonight, o'clock.*

> 8:15 a.m. *not* 8:15 a.m. o'clock
> 10:30 PM *not* 10:30 PM in the evening

Use periods with *a.m.* and *p.m.* so that *a.m.* won't be misread as the word *am*. Do not use periods with the uppercase *AM* and *PM*. Insert a space between the numerals preceding these abbreviations and the abbreviations themselves, but do not use spaces within the abbreviations.

> 11 a.m. *or* 11 AM
> *not* 11a.m. *or* 11AM
> *not* 11 a. m. *or* 11 A M

amount of

Takes a singular verb.

A minimal amount of bleeding was present.

The amount of scarring was minimal.

Amount and *number* are often confused. *Amount* refers to how much (mass), *number* to how many.

There was a small amount of bleeding, given the large number of wounds.

See number of

ampersand (&)

Symbol meaning *and*.

Use with certain single-letter abbreviations separated by *and*. Do not space before or after the ampersand. Do not use ampersand forms in operative titles or diagnoses.

D&C

T&A

D: Operation: D and C.

T: Operation: Dilatation and curettage.

Check appropriate references to identify other acceptable uses.

Some businesses use the ampersand in their name. Follow their style preferences.

Bausch & Lomb

anatomic terms

features

Do not capitalize the names of anatomic features (except the eponyms associated with them).

> os frontale
>
> zygomatic bone
>
> ligament of Treitz

posture-based terms

anterior	nearer the front
posterior	nearer the rear
superior	nearer the top
inferior	nearer the bottom

region-based terms

cranial, cephalic	nearer the head
caudal	nearer the tail or lower end
dorsal	nearer the back
ventral	nearer the belly side or anterior surface

directional and positional terms

Form directional adverbs by replacing the adjectival suffix *(-al, -or, -ic)* with the suffix *-ad*, meaning *-ward*. Use these forms in the same type of constructions in which *-ward* forms are used.

> caudad
>
> cephalad
>
> craniad
>
> laterad
>
> orad

superiad

ventrad

Do not substitute the *-ad* form when the adjective itself or the *-ly* adverb has been used correctly.

It extends caudally from...

the anterior incision

Use a combining vowel to join directional and positional adjectives.

mediolateral

Latin and English names
It is common practice to mix the English and Latin names of anatomic parts, e.g., using English for the noun and Latin for the adjectives. These may be transcribed as dictated or edited to either their English or Latin forms.

latissimus dorsi muscle

peroneus profundus nerve

palpebrales arteries

and/or

Used to indicate that one or the other or both of the items connected to it are involved. Place a virgule between the two words; do not use a hyphen.

We are considering surgery and/or chemotherapy.

and others
Latin abbreviation is *et al.* (with a period).

See Latin abbreviations

and so forth

Latin equivalent is *et ceter*a, abbreviated *etc.* Do not use *and so forth* or *etc.* when the list is preceded by *e.g.*, or *for example*.

See Latin abbreviations

angles

orthopedics

In expressing angles, write out *degrees* or use degree sign (°).

> The patient was able to straight leg raise to 40 degrees.
> *or* ...to 40°.

imaging studies

Use the degree sign (°) in imaging studies.

> Positioning the patient's head at a 90° angle allowed for efficient acquisition of data over a 180° arc.
> Coronary cineangiography was done to LAO 60°, RAO 30°.

If the symbol is not available, spell out *degree* or *degrees*.

> a 90-degree angle...a 180-degree arc
> 30-degree LAO, 30-degree cranial

electrocardiographic studies

Use the degree sign with ECG expressions related to QRS axis. If the symbol is not available, spell out *degrees*.

> QRS +60° *or* QRS +60 degrees
> A 40° LAO to 30° caudal run reveals...

APGAR questionnaire

Acronym from initial letters of **a**daptability, **p**artnership, **g**rowth, **a**ffection, **r**esolve, referring to a family assessment instrument. Use all capitals. Do not confuse with Apgar score.

Apgar score

Assessment of newborn's condition in which pulse, breathing, color, tone, and reflex irritability are each rated 0, 1, or 2, at one minute and five minutes after birth. Each set of ratings is totaled, and both totals are reported. Named after Virginia Apgar, MD.

Do not confuse with APGAR questionnaire for family assessment.

Use initial capital only.

Express ratings with arabic numerals.

Write out the numbers related to minutes, in order to avoid confusion and to draw attention to the scores.

> Apgars 7 and 9 at one and five minutes.

apostrophes

Apostrophes have many uses, the most common being to show possession, to form some plurals, and to denote omitted letters or numbers in contractions. Knowing when not to use apostrophes is as important as knowing when to use them. Medical transcription rules for apostrophes generally reflect those of common usage. Be sure to use the appropriate symbol for the apostrophe ('), if available, instead of the prime sign (').

The rules for apostrophes appear under a variety of topics throughout this book. Several are mentioned here as well.

possession

Add *'s* to show possession.

The AMA's address is...

HINT: Let pronunciation be your guide. If you would not pronounce it as *Moseses* then you would not add another *s*, just an apostrophe.

nouns ending in s

Most nouns ending in an *s* sound form the possessive, as above, with *'s*.

> Dr. Harris's patient

Often pronunciation of the possessive form is awkward when not only the last but also the next-to-last syllable ends in an *s* sound. In this case, a simple apostrophe may be more correct.

> physicians' orders
> Moses' tablets

hyphenated nouns

Use *'s* after the last word in a hyphenated compound term.

> daughter-in-law's inquiry

academic degrees

Use an apostrophe in degree designations.

> master's degree

HINT: If you can replace the possessive form with the preposition *of* without changing the meaning, the apostrophe is correct.

30 degrees' flexion =
30 degrees of flexion

5 months' pregnancy =
5 months of pregnancy

but not 5 months of pregnant
so not 5 months' pregnant

expressions of time, measurement, and money

> 20 weeks' gestation
> 30 degrees' flexion
> a few cents' worth
> a month's supply

contractions

When using contractions, take care to place the apostrophe accurately.

> The mother reported, "He's been hysterical."
> Reason for Visit: "It's time for my shot."

When referring to a single year without the century, precede it by an apostrophe.

> '99

Use a preceding apostrophe in shortened numeric expressions relating to decades of the century (his symptoms lasted all through the '90s), but omit the preceding apostrophe in expressions relating to decades of age (the patient was in his 60s).

plurals

Use 's to form the plural of lowercase abbreviations.

> *rbc's*

Use 's to form the plural of single-digit numerals or single-letter terms.

> 4 x 4's
> serial 7's

appositives

grammar

Word or phrase before or after a noun that explains or identifies it.

essential appositives

Do not use commas to set off essential, or defining, appositives (those essential to the meaning of the sentence).

Her brother Walter was tested as a potential bone marrow donor. *(The patient has more than one brother.)*

nonessential appositives

Use commas before and after nonessential (or parenthetical) appositives (those not essential to the meaning of the sentence). Sometimes other punctuation (such as parentheses or dashes) may be preferable, especially if commas cause confusion.

The surgeons, Dr. Jones and Dr. Smith, reported that the procedure was a success.

The surgeons—Dr. Jones and Dr. Smith—reported that the procedure was a success.

noun-adjective v appositive

Words that have a very close relationship are often read as a unit and no commas are needed. This can be described as a noun-adjective (a noun serving as an adjective). In the above example, *surgeons* could be seen as an adjective describing the noun-phrase *Dr. Jones and Dr. Smith*, in which case the commas would be omitted.

The surgeons Dr. Jones and Dr. Smith reported that the procedure was a success.

He accompanied his wife Alice to the clinic.

appropriate references
See references

arabic numerals
See numbers

army, Army

Capitalize when referring to a country's army; lowercase for generic references.

> The patient is a private in the US Army.
>
> They are scheduled for army physicals.
>
> There is an army of ants in his shoes.

articles

Articles *(a, an, the)* are modifiers that are used to indicate the definiteness *(the)* or indefiniteness *(a, an)* of the noun that follows. Articles are frequently dropped in dictation. They may be transcribed or not (whether dictated or not) provided their presence or absence does not substantially change the meaning or style of the originator. Articles are more apt to be included in correspondence than in reports. When dropped in transcription, it is usually because they were not dictated, they were not heard by the transcriptionist, or they were not dictated elsewhere in the report and the transcriptionist is attempting to achieve some consistency within the document.

The use of articles with abbreviations varies. Sometimes the article is required. Sometimes it is optional. Sometimes it should be omitted.

> Required: We will do a CBC.

> Optional: She was admitted to the ICU.
>
> *or* She was admitted to ICU.

> Omission required: CPR was done...
>
> *not* The CPR was done...

as

Use *as*, not *like*, as a conjunction to introduce clauses.

HINT: When using *like* or *as* to make a comparison, remember that *like* is followed by a noun and *as* is followed by a clause.

He took the medication as he was instructed.
not He took the medication like he was instructed.

as if, as though
Both are acceptable. Transcribe as dictated.

as to
Acceptable when dictated at the beginning of a sentence, but when used elsewhere, remove it or replace it by a single word, e.g., *about, in, regarding.*

As to the lab results...

He inquired [as to] whether he could drink alcohol.
(as to *can be deleted*)

D: She inquired as to the reasons for the procedure.
T: She inquired about the reasons for the procedure.

D: Her concerns as to the prognosis...
T: Her concerns regarding the prognosis...

as well as
Prepositional phrase meaning *in addition to* (equivalent to *besides*).

As well as often serves as a conjunction meaning *and in addition* (equivalent to *and*), but in either case—even when its meaning is the same as *and*—*as well as* introduces a parenthetical statement that does not create a compound subject and therefore does not affect subject-verb agreement.

The attending physician, as well as the nurses, says the patient is ready for discharge.

Use commas to set off the parenthetical *as well as* statement only as necessary for clear communication.

MRI of the brain showed right temporal contusion as well as small hemorrhagic shear in the left temporal lobe. *(no commas necessary)*

Sometimes either choice (with or without commas) is acceptable.

The patient's sister, as well as her parents, was at the meeting.
or The patient's sister as well as her parents was at the meeting.

assistant, associate

Do not abbreviate.

Do not capitalize unless used in a formal address or when part of a formal title before a name, such as in a signature line. Examples of capitalization of *assistant* and *associate* in text are rare because the terms usually represent job or occupational titles, not formal titles (even when placed before a name).

Set off with commas if the title is descriptive without the name or if the title is used to further identify the person.

The assistant surgeon, Dr. Jones, closed the wound.
or Dr. Jones, assistant surgeon, closed the wound.

Capitalize when used in a formal address or signature line.

Richard Jones, MD
Associate Professor of Clinical Psychiatry

assure, ensure, insure

While the meaning of these words is close in definition, and they all may mean *to make sure or certain*, they are not always interchangeable. *Assure* means *to make sure or certain*. It also means *to put one's mind at rest*. *Ensure* means *to make sure or certain to occur*. *Insure* may mean *to make sure or certain*, but its primary meaning is t*o issue or obtain insurance in order to guarantee persons or property against risk*.

> Be assured that this disease is not fatal.
>
> Visiting nurses will ensure that the patient takes his medications.
>
> The patient has health insurance with her employer, but she wanted to know how she could insure her children as well.

audit trails

Also known as documentation trails, audit trails contribute to risk management. An audit trail is simply a careful sequential record of actions and conversations on a particular matter. This type of record is recommended for any event considered legally sensitive, including circumstances where medical transcriptionists are advised or directed to act contrary to usual practices or legal directives.

autopsy report

Report prepared by a pathologist or medical examiner to document findings on examination of a cadaver. Typical content topics include medical history, course of treatment, external and internal examinations, evidence of injury, macroscopic and microscopic examinations, gross findings (systems and organs), special dissections, pathologic diagnosis, and cause of death.

See Appendix A: Sample Reports

average of

This phrase takes a plural verb if preceded by *an*, singular if preceded by *the*.

> An average of 10 tests were done on each patient.
>
> The average of the results was 48.3%.

B

bachelor's degree

Lowercase and use the possessive with this generic form. Use capitals only when it follows a person's name. Note: The term *degree* is always lowercase.

> He has a bachelor's degree in engineering.
>
> The patient has a bachelor of arts degree.
>
> Jane Smith, Bachelor of Fine Arts

See degrees, academic

back formations

See language to avoid

basic fundamental

Since the two words have the same meaning, the phrase is redundant. Use one word or the other.

> The basic problem was...
>
> *or* The fundamental problem was...
>
> *not* The basic fundamental problem was...

bay, Bay

Capitalize when integral to a proper name and in popular names that are widely used and accepted; otherwise, lowercase.

> Morro Bay
> Chesapeake Bay
> the Bay Area
> He walked along the bay.

bc, bcc

See copy designation

beats per minute

Commonly abbreviated *BPM* or *bpm*.

> Pulse: 70 beats per minute.
> *or* Pulse: 70 BPM.
> *or* Pulse: 70 bpm.

because, due to, since

The following usage delineations are becoming more and more blurred, and these terms can generally be transcribed as dictated.

because

Means *for the reason that*. Denotes a specific cause-effect relationship.

> He has been in pain because his arm was broken.

due to

Means *caused by* or *resulting from*, not *because*.

> Her reaction was due to a penicillin allergy.
> *not* Her reaction was because of a penicillin allergy.

> She was late because her watch stopped.
> *not* She was late due to her watch stopping.

Due to is properly used after a linking verb (*was* due to), but the verb may be omitted in an elliptical clause.

> His complications, though due to negligence, were not life-threatening.

since

When it introduces a clause not set off by a comma or when it is used as a preposition, *since* means *after the time that*, indicating that an event follows another but was not caused by it.

> He has been in pain since he returned from vacation.

Since means *because* when it introduces a clause set off by a comma.

> He has omitted his rofecoxib for the past 3 weeks, since it was upsetting his stomach.

b.i.d.

See drug terminology

bilateral

Adjective that may modify either a plural or a singular noun, depending upon the meaning.

bilateral decision *(A decision made by people on both [usually opposing] sides of an issue acting together.)*

bilateral pneumonia *(There is only one condition, although present in both lungs at the same time.)*

bilateral mastectomies *(There are two breasts and both are removed, so it's plural.)*

bilateral tympanostomies and Teflon tube insertions

 biopsy

The use of this noun as a verb is common in medical dictation. Transcribe as dictated.

The liver was biopsied.
or A biopsy of the liver was done.

 black

Both *African American* and *black* are acceptable designations for Americans of African heritage. (Most publications lowercase all designations of race and ethnicity based on color, although some capitalize *Black*.)

The patient is a 35-year-old black man.

See sociocultural designations

blank

See dictation problems

blood counts

differential blood count

Part of a white blood cell count. Includes polymorphonuclear neutrophils (PMNs, polys, segmented neutrophils [segs]), band neutrophils (bands, stabs), lymphocytes (lymphs), eosinophils (eos), basophils (basos), and monocytes (monos).

Differential counts may be given as whole numbers or as percents; total should equal 100 in either case.

> White blood count of 4800, with 58% segs, 7% bands, 24% lymphs, 8% monos, 1% eos, and 2% basos.
>
> *or* White blood count of 4800, with 58 segs, 7 bands, 24 lymphs, 8 monos, 1 eo, and 2 basos.

RBC, rbc

Either form is acceptable as an abbreviation for red blood count or red blood cells.

WBC, wbc

Either form is acceptable as an abbreviation for white blood count or white blood cells.

white blood count

See differential blood count *above*.

blood groups

ABO system

Use single or dual letters, sometimes with a subscript letter or number. If subscripts are not available, place the numeral immediately following and on the line with the letter.

> group A
> group A1 or group A_1
> group A1B or group A_1B

other systems

Other common blood group systems include Auberger, Diego, Duffy, Kell, Kidd, Lewis, Lutheran, Rh (not *Rhesus*), Sutter, and Xg. Consult laboratory references for guidance in expressing terms related to these and other blood groups.

blood pressure (BP)
abbreviated form

Often abbreviated *BP*.

> D: Blood pressure 110/80.
> T: Blood pressure 110/80.
> *or* BP 110/80.

blood pressure ranges

> D: Blood pressure was 100 to 120 over 70 to 80.
> T: Blood pressure was 100-120 over 70-80.
> *or* ...100 to 120 over 70 to 80.
> *or* Blood pressure was in the 100-120 over 70-80 range.

Not acceptable because they may be misunderstood are:

> 100-120/70-80
> *and* 100/70 to 120/80

use of mmHg

Blood pressure is reported in *mmHg*, but often only the values are dictated. Do not delete *mmHg* if dictated. It may be added if not dictated.

> D: Blood pressure 110/80.
> T: Blood pressure 110/80.
> *or* Blood pressure 110/80 mmHg.

blood types

Write out *B negative* or *B positive* rather than *B-* or *B+*, because the minus or plus sign is easily overlooked.

body cavities

Body spaces containing internal organs.

cavity	organs
cranial	brain
thoracic	esophagus, trachea, thymus gland, aorta, lungs, heart
abdominal	gallbladder, liver, spleen, pancreas, stomach, small intestine, large intestine
pelvic	urinary bladder, urethra, ureters (in female: uterus and vagina, as well)
spinal	nerves of spinal cord

body parts

Phrases such as *left heart* and *right chest* are frequently dictated when what is meant is left side of heart, right side of chest. These phrases may be transcribed as dictated unless their usage would confuse or amuse rather than communicate.

left heart catheterization

right chest abscess

left neck incision

both

Use *both*, when dictated, to refer to two items. Delete the word *both* if more than two items follow.

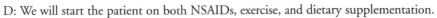

D: We will start the patient on both NSAIDs, exercise, and dietary supplementation.

T: We will start the patient on NSAIDs, exercise, and dietary supplementation.

braces { }

Braces are commonly used in chemical nomenclature and mathematical formulas.

See chemical nomenclature

 brackets [ ]

Brackets are commonly used in chemical nomenclature and mathematical formulas. They are also used to delineate a parenthetical insertion within parenthetical material. An originator will often dictate "brackets" when *parentheses* is meant. Use parentheses unless it is truly a parenthetical insertion within parenthetical material.

See chemical nomenclature
    parentheses

 bring, take

Bring is generally used to signify movement toward and *take*, movement away from. However, switching the usage of these terms is also considered grammatical. Transcribe as dictated.

British spelling

Some terms are spelled differently in the United States than in Great Britain and other English-speaking countries such as Canada and Australia. Use the form that is preferred in the country for which you are transcribing.

American	British
aluminum	aluminium
cecum	caecum
celiac	coeliac
center	centre
esophagus	oesophagus
fiber	fibre
honor	honour

meter	metre
orthopedic	orthopaedic
pediatric	paediatric

Some British spellings are used in official names in the United States, and in those cases the preferred spelling of that business or organization should be used.

American Academy of Orthopaedics

British thermal unit (BTU)

Use abbreviation *BTU* with arabic numerals. Use same form for singular or plural.

1 BTU
4 BTU

Brown and Sharp gauge

See suture sizes

bruit

An abnormal heart sound or murmur heard on auscultation. The plural form is *bruits* but because of the French origin of the word, often the final *s* is not pronounced and the singular and plural sound the same: "broo-ee."

building, structure, and room names

Capitalize proper names of office buildings, government buildings, churches, hospitals, hotels. Do not abbreviate. Capitalize the word *building* or similar words only if they are an integral part of the official name.

the White House
Memorial Hospital
but the Damrell building

Capitalize proper names of structures, monuments, etc. Lowercase generic terms.

> She fell while visiting the Tomb of the Unknown Soldier.
> He tripped on the steps of the Capitol.
> She fell against the Rodin sculpture.

Capitalize names of specially designated rooms only.

> She attended a reception in the Rose Room at the White House.
> The patient will be seen in 3 weeks in Dr. Smith's Limb Deficiency Clinic.

Do not capitalize common nouns designating rooms; these are generic terms applied to all similar rooms.

> He was admitted through the emergency room.
> She left the operating room in good condition.

Use abbreviations for room names only if dictated **and** if they will be readily recognized by the reader.

> He was admitted to the ICU.
> *or* He was admitted to the intensive care unit.

Use arabic numerals for room numbers. Lowercase *room*.

> The patient is in room 148.

Capitalize all elements of a building address, including the room name.

> Sister Mary Helene
> St. Agnes Hospital Emergency Room
> Ourtown, USA

bur, burr

A rotary cutting instrument or drill. The preferred medical spelling is *bur*.

burn classifications

See classification systems

business names

Express according to the business's style and usage. Use the full name before using the abbreviated form in order to avoid confusion among similar abbreviations except for businesses, such as IBM, that are better known by their abbreviations than by their full names.

In general, use initial caps for all words in a business name except articles and prepositions or words that the business chooses to lowercase.

> eBay

Capitalize words such as *organization, institution, association* only when they are part of the entity's official name; do not capitalize them when they are used alone or in a shortened version of the name. Note: The entity, in shortened references to itself, may choose to use initial capitals.

> American Hospital Association
> *but* the association
> *or* the hospital association

abbreviations/acronyms

Some businesses are readily recognized by their abbreviations or acronyms and may be referred to by same if dictated and if there is reasonable assurance the business will be accurately identified by the reader. Most abbreviated forms use all capitals and do not use periods, but be guided by the entity's designated abbreviated form.

> IBM equipment
> He is an ACLU attorney.

ampersand

Use an ampersand *(&)* in a company, corporation, or partnership name when it is part of that entity's formal expression of its name. In these instances, space before and after the ampersand if it separates words or multiple letters; do not space if it separates single letters. Exception: If the entity does not use spaces with the ampersand, follow the entity's style choice.

> Bausch & Lomb
> AT&T
> C&H Sugar

company, Company

Capitalize *company* only if part of an official name.

> Campbell Soup Company
> company policy

Co., Corp., Inc., Ltd.

Abbreviate and capitalize *Co., Corp., Inc.,* or *Ltd.* only when the business being named uses the abbreviation in its formal name. Do not use a comma before *Inc.* or *Ltd.* unless the specific entity uses it.

> Ford Motor Co.

Form possessive of names using abbreviation *Co., Corp., Inc.,* or *Ltd.,* as follows:

> Ford Motor Co.'s annual report

departments

Lowercase common nouns designating department names; reserve capitals for proper nouns or adjectives, in addresses, or when part of a federal government agency name.

She is head of the St. Mary's Hospital surgery department.

He works for the State Department in Washington, DC.

The patient is head of the English department at the local state university.

However, capitalize a department name that is referred to as an entity.

The patient was referred to Anesthesia for preoperative evaluation.

The report from Pathology indicates that the tumor is benign.

divisions

Lowercase common nouns naming institutional divisions.

the administrative division of Memorial Hospital

internal units

Lowercase common names for internal units of an organization.

The patient's medication was changed because apparently the pharmacy can no longer obtain paregoric.

Exception: Capitalization may be used for such internal units in the entity's references to itself in its own formal and/or legal documents.

Please note the change in Pharmacy hours...

Capitalize internal elements when their names are not generic terms.

Dr. Smith's Limb Deficiency Clinic

inverted forms

When inverted forms of names are widely used and recognized, capitalize those forms as well.

> College of William and Mary
> William and Mary College

businessperson

Generic, nonsexist form, preferred to *businessman* and *businesswoman*.

See sexist language

but meaning only

When *but* is used to mean *only*, it is a negative and should not be preceded by *not*.

> D: She was not seen but once.
> T: She was seen but once.

by

See X, x

C

c, C, c

The abbreviation *c* is for *copy* and *C* is for *Celsius*.

The medical symbol $\bar{c}$ meaning *with* is frequently used in handwritten notes. Do not use $\bar{c}$ in transcribed reports; use *with* instead.

caliber of weapons

Express with decimal point followed by arabic numerals and a hyphen. Do not place a zero before the decimal point.

> .38-caliber pistol

Canada

Canadian territories and provinces

Capitalize full names of Canadian territories.

> Northwest Territories
> Yukon Territory

Use commas to set off community names from names of provinces. Do not capitalize *province*. Do not abbreviate names of provinces in reports.

> She is from Toronto, Ontario. (*not* Toronto, Ont.)
> the province of Ontario

French Canadian

Do not hyphenate.

C

cancer classifications
stage and grade
Lowercase *stage* and *grade*.

Use roman numerals for cancer stages. For subdivisions of cancer stages, add capital letters on the line and arabic suffixes, without internal spaces or hyphens.

> stage 0 *(indicates carcinoma in situ)*
> stage I, stage IA
> stage II, stage II3
> stage III
> stage IV, stage IVB

Use arabic numerals for grades.

> grade 1
> grade 2
> grade 3
> grade 4

Aster-Coller
Staging system for colon cancer from the least involvement at stage A and B1 through the most extensive involvement at stage D.

> The patient's Aster-Coller B2 lesion extends through the entire thickness of the colon wall, with no involvement of nearby nodes.

Broders index
Classification of aggressiveness of tumor malignancy developed in the 1920s by AC Broders. Reported as grade 1 (most differentiation and best prognosis) through grade 4 (least differentiation and poorest prognosis).

C

Lowercase *grade*; use arabic numerals.

> Broders grade 3

cervical cytology

Three different systems are currently in use for cervical cytology: the Papanicolaou test (Pap smear), the CIN classification system, and the Bethesda system.

The Papanicolaou test uses roman numerals to classify cervical cytology samples from class I (within normal limits) through class V (carcinoma).

CIN is an acronym for *cervical intraepithelial neoplasia* and is expressed with arabic numerals from grade 1 (least severe) to grade 3 (most severe). Place a hyphen between *CIN* and the numeral.

> CIN-1, CIN-2, CIN-3
> *or* CIN grade 1, CIN grade 2, CIN grade 3

A cervical cytology sample that is within normal limits in the Bethesda system corresponds with a Pap class I or II; Bethesda's atypical squamous cell of undetermined significance (ASCUS) corresponds with Pap class III; Bethesda's low-grade squamous intraepithelial lesion (LGSIL) corresponds with Pap class III and CIN grade 1; and Bethesda's high-grade squamous intraepithelial lesion (HGSIL) corresponds with Pap classes III and IV and CIN grades 2 and 3. In the Bethesda system, the next higher level is labeled simply "carcinoma," corresponding with Pap class V and with "carcinoma" in the CIN system.

Clark level

Describes invasion level of primary malignant melanoma of the skin from the epidermis.

C

Use roman numerals I (least deep) to IV (deepest). Lowercase *level*.

Clark level I	into underlying papillary dermis
Clark level II	to junction of papillary and reticular dermis
Clark level III	into reticular dermis
Clark level IV	into the subcutaneous fat

Dukes classification

Named for British pathologist Cuthbert E. Dukes (1890-1977). Classifies extent of operable adenocarcinoma of the colon or rectum.

Do not use an apostrophe before or after the *s*. Follow *Dukes* with capital letter.

Dukes A	confined to mucosa
Dukes B	extending into the muscularis mucosae
Dukes C	extending through the bowel wall, with metastasis to lymph nodes

When the Dukes classification is further defined by numbers, use arabic numerals on the same line with the letter, with no space between.

Dukes C2

FAB classification

French-**A**merican-**B**ritish morphologic classification system for acute nonlymphoid leukemia.

Express with capital *M* followed by arabic numeral (1 through 6); do not space between the *M* and the numeral.

M1	myeloblastic, no differentiation
M2	myeloblastic, differentiation

M3	promyelocytic
M4	myelomonocytic
M5	monocytic
M6	erythroleukemia

FAB staging of carcinoma utilizes TNM classification of malignant tumors (*See* TNM staging *below*).

FAB T1 N1 M0

FIGO staging

Federation **I**nternationale de **G**ynécologie et **O**bstétrique system for staging gynecologic malignancy, particularly carcinomas of the ovary. Expressed as stage I (least severe) to stage IV (most severe), with subdivisions within each stage (a, b, c).

Lowercase *stage*, and use roman numerals. Use lowercase letters to indicate subdivisions within a stage.

Diagnosis: Ovarian carcinoma, FIGO stage IIc.

Gleason tumor grade

Also known as Gleason score. The system scores or grades the prognosis for adenocarcinoma of the prostate, with a scale of 1 through 5 for each dominant and secondary pattern; these are then totaled for the score. The higher the score, the poorer the prognosis.

Lowercase *grade* or *score*, and use arabic numerals.

Diagnosis: Adenocarcinoma of prostate, Gleason score 8.
Gleason score 3 + 2 = 5.
Gleason 3 + 3 with a total score of 6.

Jewett classification of bladder carcinoma
Use capitals as follows:

O   in situ (*Note: this is the letter* O, *not a zero*)
A   involving submucosa
B   involving muscle
C   involving surrounding tissue
D   involving distant sites

Diagnosis: Bladder carcinoma, Jewett class B.

Karnofsky rating scale, Karnofsky status
Scale for rating performance status of patients with malignant neoplasms.

Use arabic numerals: 10, 20, 30, 40, 50, 60, 70, 80, 90, 100. (Normal is 100, moribund is 10.)

TNM staging system for malignant tumors
System for staging malignant tumors, developed by the American Joint Committee on Cancer and the Union Internationale Contre le Cancer.

T   **t**umor size or involvement
N   regional lymph **n**ode involvement
M   extent of **m**etastasis

Write TNM expressions with arabic numerals on the line and a space after each number.

T2 N1 M1
T4 N3 M1

Letters and symbols following the letters *T, N,* and *M*:

> *X* means assessment cannot be done.
>
> *0 (zero)* indicates no evidence found.
>
> Numbers indicate increasing evidence of the characteristics represented by those letters.
>
> *Tis* indicates tumor in situ.

Tis N0 M0

The TNM system criteria for defining cancer stages vary according to the type of cancer. Thus a stage II cancer of one type may be defined as T1 N0 M0, while one of another type may be defined as T2 N1 M0.

Staging indicators are used along with TNM criteria to define cancers and assess stages. These are expressed with capital letters and arabic numerals.

grade	GX, G1, G2, G3, G4
host performance	H0, H1, H2, H3, H4
lymphatic invasion	LX, L0, L1, L2
residual tumor	RX, R0, R1, R2
scleral invasion	SX, S0, S1, S2
venous invasion	VX, V0, V1, V2

prefixes

Lowercase prefixes on the line with TNM and other symbols indicate criteria used to describe and stage the tumor, e.g., cTNM, aT2.

letter	*determining criteria*
a	autopsy staging
c	clinical classification
p	pathological classification
r	retreatment classification
y, yp	classification during or following treatment with multiple modalities

C

suffixes

The suffix *(m)* (in parentheses) indicates the presence of multiple primary tumors in a single site. Other suffixes may be used, such as the following in the nasopharynx:

T2a   nasopharyngeal tumor extending to soft tissues of oropharynx and/or nasal fossa *without* parapharyngeal extension

T2b   nasopharyngeal tumor extending to soft tissues of oropharynx and/or nasal fossa *with* parapharyngeal extension

cannot, can't

Use *cannot* instead of *can not*.

Use *cannot* instead of shortened form *can't* except in direct quotations.

See contractions

capitalization

Capitals emphasize and draw attention to the terms in which they are used. Use them appropriately and judiciously because their overuse diminishes their value and impact.

Some words are always capitalized, some never. The placement or use of a term may determine whether it is capitalized. Capitals, for example, are always used to mark the beginning of a sentence.

Learning and adopting the rules of capitalization, when they should be used and when they should not be used, as well as the few instances when variations may be acceptable, will improve the consistency, accuracy, and communication value of transcribed healthcare documents.

In particular, avoid the use of unnecessary or inappropriate capitals. Do not, for example, capitalize a common-noun reference to a thing or person if it is just one of many other such things or persons. Thus, *emergency room* and *recovery room* are not capitalized. Think of the rule for generic versus brand names for drugs. The generic term (common noun) *emergency room* is applied to all emergency rooms, so it is not capitalized.

cardiology

EKG terms

ECG and *EKG* are acceptable abbreviations for *electrocardiogram, electrocardiography, electrocardiographic.* Transcribe as dictated.

leads

Electronic connections for recording by means of electrocardiograph. Where subscripts are called for but are not available, standard-size numerals and letters on the line may be used.

standard bipolar leads: Use roman numerals.

lead I, lead II, lead III

augmented limb leads: Use a lowercase *a* followed by a capital *V*, then a capital *R* (right), *L* (left), or *F* (foot).

aVR, aVL, aVF

precordial leads: Use a capital *V* followed by an arabic numeral. Enter the numeral in the same point size on the line with the *V*, with no space between, or use subscripting.

V1, V2, V3, V4, V5, V6, V7, V8, V9
or V_1, V_2, V_3, V_4, V_5, V_6, V_7, V_8, V_9

right precordial leads: Use a capital *V* followed by an arabic numeral and capital *R*. Enter the numeral and *R* in the same point size on the line with the *V*, with no space between, or use subscripting.

> V3R, V4R, etc.
> *or* V_3R, V_4R, etc.

ensiform cartilage lead: Use a capital *V* followed by a capital *E* in the same point size on the line with the *V*, with no space between, or subscript the *E*.

> VE *or* V_E

third interspace leads: Use an arabic numeral followed by capital *V* and an arabic numeral. Enter the numeral following the *V* as a subscript or in the same point size on the line, with no space between.

> 3V1, 3V2, 3V3, etc.
> *or* $3V_1$, $3V_2$, $3V_3$, etc.

esophageal leads: Use a capital *E* followed by an arabic numeral either subscripted or on the line in the same point size, with no space between.

> E15, E24, E50, etc.
> *or* E_{15}, E_{24}, E_{50}, etc.

sequential leads: Repeat the *V*. Do not use a hyphen or dash.

> leads V1 through V5 *or* V_1 through V_5
> *not* V1 through 5 *or* V_1 through $_5$
> *not* V1-V5 *or* V_1-V_5
> *not* V1-5 *or* V_{1-5}

tracing terms

In general, for electrocardiographic deflections, use all capitals, but larger and smaller Q, R, and S waves may be differentiated by capital and lowercase letters, respectively. Do not place a hyphen after the single letter except when the term is used as an adjective.

> Q wave, q wave
>
> QS wave, qs wave
>
> R wave, r wave
>
> S wave, s wave
>
> R' wave, r' wave (*Note:* R' *is dictated as* "R prime")
>
> S' wave, s' wave

For terms such as *P wave*, in which there is no hyphen, insert a hyphen when the term is used as an adjective *(P-wave pathology)*.

> J junction
>
> J point
>
> P wave
>
> QT interval, prolongation, etc.
>
> QT_c (*if subscript is not available, express as* QTc *or* corrected QT interval)
>
> PR interval, segment, etc.
>
> QRS axis, complex, configuration, etc.
>
> ST segment
>
> ST-T elevation
>
> T wave
>
> T-wave abnormality
>
> Ta wave
>
> U wave

For *QRS axis*, use a plus or a minus sign followed by arabic numerals and a degree sign to express the number of degrees, e.g., QRS +60°, or write out *degrees*: QRS +60 degrees.

heart sounds and murmurs

Abbreviate heart sounds and components as follows, placing numerals on the line or using subscripts.

first heart sound	S1 *or* S_1
second heart sound	S2 *or* S_2
third heart sound	S3 *or* S_3
fourth heart sound	S4 *or* S_4
aortic valve component	A2 *or* A_2
mitral valve component	M1 *or* M_1
pulmonic valve component	P2 *or* P_2
tricuspid valve component	T1 *or* T_1

Express murmurs with arabic numerals 1 to 6 (from soft or low-grade to loud or high-grade). Do not use roman numerals. Murmurs are expressed on either a scale of 1 to 4 or a scale of 1 to 6. The scale of 6 breaks down as follows:

grade 1	barely audible, must strain to hear
grade 2	quiet, but clearly audible
grade 3	moderately loud
grade 4	loud
grade 5	very loud; audible with stethoscope partly off the chest
grade 6	so loud that it can be heard with stethoscope just above chest wall

Place a virgule between the murmur grade and the scale used (2/4 = a grade 2 murmur on a scale of 4).

grade 1/6 systolic murmur

Express partial units as indicated.

D: grade 4 and a half over 6 murmur
T: grade 4.5 over 6 murmur
or grade 4.5/6 murmur

D: grade 4 to 5 over 6 murmur
T: grade 4 to 5 over 6 murmur
or grade 4/6 to 5/6 murmur
not grade 4-5/6 murmur

D: to-and-fro SDM
T: to-and-fro systolic-diastolic murmur

A bruit is an abnormal heart sound or murmur heard on auscultation. The plural form is *bruits* but because of the French origin of the word, often the final *s* is not pronounced and the singular and plural forms sound the same: "broo-ee."

Spell out the following abbreviations even when they are dictated in phonocardiographic tracings.

ASM	atrial systolic murmur	AEC	aortic ejection click
CM	continuous murmur	AOC	aortic opening click
DM	diastolic murmur	C	click
DSM	delayed systolic murmur	E	ejection sound
ESM	ejection systolic murmur	EC	ejection click
IDM	immediate diastolic murmur	NEC	nonejection click
LSM	late systolic murmur	PEC	pulmonary ejection click
PSM	pansystolic murmur	OS	opening snap
SDM	systolic-diastolic murmur	SC	systolic click
SEM	systolic ejection murmur	SS	summation sound
SM	systolic murmur	W	whoop

C

NYHA classification of cardiac failure

Widely adopted classification of cardiac failure that was developed by the **N**ew **Y**ork **H**eart **A**ssociation. Lowercase *class*; use roman numerals *I* through *IV*.

I	asymptomatic
II	comfortable at rest, symptomatic with normal activity
III	comfortable at rest, symptomatic with less than normal activity
IV	severe cardiac failure, symptomatic at rest

DIAGNOSIS: Cardiac failure, class III.

pacemaker codes

Capitalize these three-letter codes, without spaces or periods.

AVD
ITR

First and second letters refer to

A	atrium
V	ventricle
D	dual, both atrium and ventricle

Third letter refers to

I	inhibited response
T	triggered response
R	rate-responsive response

TIMI system

Thrombolysis **i**n **m**yocardial **i**nfarction. A grading system (grade 0 to 3) for coronary perfusion; evaluates reperfusion achieved by thrombolytic therapy. Lowercase *grade* and use arabic numerals.

The patient had TIMI grade 3 flow at 90 minutes following thrombolytic therapy.

Caucasian, white

Always capitalize *Caucasian*.

> This is a 59-year-old Caucasian woman.

Unless it begins a sentence, *white* is not capitalized.

> This is a 59-year-old white woman.

cc

Abbreviation for *courtesy copy* or *carbon copy*. Do not use periods.

Note: Instead of *cc* for *cubic centimeters*, which is on the ISMP list of dangerous abbreviations, use the equivalent *mL (milliliter)*, which is the preferred term.

See Appendix B: Dangerous Abbreviations

Centers for Medicare and Medicaid Services (CMS)

The bureau of the US Department of Health and Human Services that administers federal Medicare and Medicaid programs. Until 2001 it was called the Health Care Financing Administration (HCFA). Note that *Centers* ends in *s* but takes a singular verb.

Centers for Disease Control and Prevention (CDC)

An agency of the US Department of Health and Human Services whose mission is to promote health and quality of life by preventing and controlling disease, injury, and disability. Note that *Centers* ends in *s* but takes a singular verb.

C

centi-

Inseparable prefix denoting one-hundredth of a unit. To convert to basic unit, move decimal point two places to the left.

> 256 centimeters = 2.56 meters

Use decimals, not fractions, with metric units of measure when possible.

> D: two and a half centimeters
> T: 2.5 cm

Occasionally, the originator will use a fraction that cannot be exactly translated into decimals. In such cases, transcribe as dictated.

> D: three and two thirds centimeters
> T: 3-2/3 cm

centigrade

See temperature, temperature scales

centigray (cGy)

One-hundredth of a gray, the SI (International System of Units) unit of absorbed dose of ionizing radiation.

Abbreviation: *cGy* (no periods).

centimeter (cm)

One-hundredth of a meter. Also equal to 10 millimeters. To convert to inches, multiply by 0.4.

Abbreviation: cm (no period).

160 cm = 64 inches

certified medical transcriptionist (CMT)

Professional designation awarded to individuals who have met certification requirements as specified by the Medical Transcription Certification Commission at AAMT.

Use capital letters for the abbreviation. Do not use periods. Lowercase the extended form unless it follows a person's name as in the following example.

James Morrison, Certified Medical Transcriptionist
CMT
She is a certified medical transcriptionist

Do not link *CMT* to another professional or academic designation by a virgule or hyphen; rather, place a comma and space between them.

Jo Workman, CMT, RHIT *not* Jo Workman, CMT/RHIT

Do not use *CMT* after the personal initials for a transcriptionist. (Likewise, do not add *MD* or other professional designations or academic degrees to an originator's initials.)

db:jb *not* db:jbcmt *not* dbmd:jbcmt

Do not use the abbreviations *MT* (medical transcriptionist) or *MLS* (medical language specialist) after one's name because doing so gives the impression it carries the weight of a professional certification designation. *CMT* is the only recognized professional certification designation for medical transcriptionists, and it may be used only if authorized through the Medical Transcription Certification Commission at AAMT.

C

Note: Other certifications that may be designated by the abbreviation *CMT* include *certified massage therapist* and *certified music therapist*.

cervical intraepithelial neoplasia

Abbreviation: *CIN* (no periods).

See cancer classifications

cesarean section, C-section

See obstetrics terminology

chair, chairperson

Generic, nonsexist term, preferred to *chairman* or *chairwoman*.

character spacing

When using a proportional-spaced font it is customary to mark the end of a sentence with a single space; however, double-spacing is still widely used, especially with non-proportional fonts, such as Courier. The choice is usually determined by departmental or company policy.

Use either a single character space or two spaces (but be consistent in your usage) **after**

- the end of a sentence, whether it ends in a period, question mark, exclamation point, quotation mark, parenthesis, bracket, or brace
- a colon used as a punctuation mark within a sentence

Use a single character space **after**

- each word or symbol (unless the next character is a punctuation mark)
- a comma

- a semicolon
- a period at the end of an abbreviation

Use a single character space **before**

- an opening quotation mark
- an opening parenthesis
- an opening bracket or brace

Do not use a character space **before or after**

- an apostrophe (except when the apostrophe ends the term, as in the plural possessive *patients',* in which case a space or another punctuation mark follows the apostrophe)
- a colon in expressions of time or clock or equator positions, e.g., 1:30
- a colon in expressions of ratios and dilutions, e.g., 1:100,000
- a comma in numeric expressions, e.g., 12,034
- a decimal point in numeric expressions (except in those rare instances when a unit less than 1 does not call for a zero to be placed before the decimal, e.g., .22-caliber rifle, in which instances a space precedes the decimal point but does not follow it)
- a decimal point in monetary expressions, e.g., $1.50
- a hyphen, e.g., 3-0 suture material
- a dash, e.g.: Episodes of dyspnea—usually without pain—occur on slight exertion.
- a virgule, e.g., 2/6 heart murmur
- a period within an abbreviation, e.g., q.i.d.
- an ampersand in abbreviations such as T&A, D&C

Do not use a character space **after**

- an opening quotation mark
- an opening parenthesis, bracket, or brace
- a word followed by a punctuation mark

C

Do not use a character space **before**

• a punctuation mark (except an opening parenthesis, bracket, brace, or quotation mark)

chemical nomenclature
elements and symbols

Names of elements are not capitalized. The symbols for chemical elements always include an initial capital letter; if there is a second letter, it is always lowercase. Never use periods or other punctuation with chemical symbols.

The following is a list of some of the more commonly encountered elements from the periodic table, with their symbols.

barium	Ba	gallium	Ga	nitrogen	N
calcium	Ca	gold	Au	oxygen	O
carbon	C	hydrogen	H	potassium	K
cesium	Cs	iodine	I	silver	Ag
chlorine	Cl	iron	Fe	sodium	Na
cobalt	Co	lead	Pb	sulfur	S
copper	Cu	magnesium	Mg	technetium	Tc
gadolinium	Gd	mercury	Hg	zinc	Zn

compounds

Lowercase the names of chemical compounds written in full.

Never use hyphens in chemical elements or compounds, whether used as nouns or adjectives.

carbon dioxide
potassium
carbon monoxide poisoning

chemical names

Do not capitalize chemical names, except at the beginning of a sentence.

> acetylsalicylic acid
> oxygen

concentration

Use brackets to express chemical concentration. When concentrations are expressed as percentages, use the percent sign rather than the spelled-out form and do not use brackets.

> [HCO3$^-$] *or* [HCO$_3^-$]
> 15% HNO3 *or* HNO$_3$

formulas

Use parentheses for innermost units, adding brackets, then braces, if necessary. (Note that this is different from regular text, which uses brackets for the innermost parenthetical insertion and parentheses for the outermost.) Italics may also be used for some portions; consult chemistry references. Two examples of chemical formulas follow.

> chlorphenoxamine hydrochloride
> 2-[1-(4-chlorophenyl)-1-phenylethoxy]-*N,N*-dimethylethanamine hydrochloride

> hydroxychloroquine sulfate
> 7-chloro-4-{4-[ethyl(2-hydroxyethyl)amino]-1-methylbutylamino}-quinoline sulfate

biochemical terminology

Write out biochemical terms in healthcare documents because their abbreviations may not be readily recognized by healthcare professionals.

Use abbreviated forms only in tables and in communications among biochemical specialists.

C

examples of biochemical groups, terms, and abbreviations
(3-letter and/or 1-letter)

amino acids of proteins	phenylalanine	Phe, F
	proline	Pro, P
	tryptophan	Trp, W
bases and nucleosides	cytosine	Cyt
	purine	Pur
	uracil	Ura
common ribonucleosides	adenosine	Ado, A
	cytidine	Cyd, C
	uridine	Urd, U
sugars and carbohydrates	fructose	Fru
	glucose	Rib

Chicana, Chicano

Usage and acceptance of this designation for a Mexican American is preferred by some, considered derogatory by others. Use *Chicana* for female, *Chicano* for male. Plural form: *Chicanos*. A widely preferred alternative to *Chicana/Chicano* is *Mexican American* or *Hispanic*. Transcribe whatever term is dictated.

See sociocultural designations

chief, Chief

Capitalize only if it is a formal title and it precedes a name; otherwise, lowercase.

Chief Watson

The chief called an emergency meeting.

Child classification of hepatic risk criteria

See classification systems

chromosomal terms

See genetics

church, Church

Capitalize only when part of the proper name of an organization, building, congregation, or denomination; otherwise, lowercase.

> St. Mary's Church
>
> Cornerstone Baptist Church
>
> the neighborhood church

Clark level

See cancer classifications

classification systems

Systematic arrangements into groups or classes. *See also* cancer classifications, cardiology, obstetrics, *and* orthopedics.

Some classification systems use arabic numerals and others call for roman. In some systems there is no agreement on the use of roman versus arabic numerals. There is a trend away from the use of roman numerals, and generally speaking, the preference is for using arabic numerals unless it is documented that roman numerals are required. Several classification systems are listed below; check appropriate references for additional guidance.

Apgar score

Assessment of newborn's condition in which pulse, breathing, color, tone, and reflex irritability are each rated 0, 1, or 2, at one minute and five minutes after birth. Each set of ratings is totaled, and both totals are reported. Named after Virginia Apgar, MD.

Do not confuse with APGAR questionnaire for family assessment.

Use initial capital only.

Express ratings with arabic numerals.

Write out the numbers related to minutes, so that attention is drawn to the scores and confusion is avoided.

> Apgars 7 and 9 at one and five minutes.

Ballard scale
A scoring system for assessing the gestational age of infants based on neuromuscular and physical maturity. Scores are converted to gestational age (in weeks).

Express in arabic numerals.

score	age (weeks)
5	26
10	28
15	30
20	32
25	34
30	36
35	38
40	40
45	42
50	44

burn classifications
Burns are described as 1st, 2nd, 3rd, and 4th degree, according to burn depth.

AAMT recommends dropping the hyphen in the adjective form (e.g., 1st degree burn), though use of the hyphen is acceptable.

Expressing ordinals as numerals is preferred to writing them out: 1st, 2nd,

3rd, and 4th degree burns, not first, second, third, and fourth degree burns.

Rule of Nines: Formula, based on multiples of 9, for determining percentage of burned body surface. This formula does not apply to children because a child's head is disproportionately large.

head	9%
each arm	9%
each leg	18%
anterior trunk	18%
posterior trunk	18%
perineum	1%

Berkow formula: Rule of Nines adjusted for a patient's age. Assigns a higher percentage to a child's head, which is larger than an adult's head in proportion to its body.

Catterall hip score

Rating system for Legg-Perthes disease (pediatric avascular necrosis of the femoral head).

Use roman numerals I (no findings) through IV (involvement of entire femoral head).

Child classification of hepatic risk criteria

Classification of operative risk.

Capitalize *Child* (eponymic term), lowercase *class*, and capitalize the letter that follows.

Child class A
Child class B
Child class C

decubitus ulcers

Decubitus ulcers are classified using roman numerals from stage I (nonblanchable erythema of intact skin) through stage IV (full-thickness skin loss with extensive tissue destruction).

diabetes mellitus classifications

See diabetes mellitus

Epworth Sleepiness Scale

Measures daytime sleepiness on a scale of 1 to 24. Use arabic numerals.

> Less than 8: Normal sleep function
> 8-10: Mild sleepiness
> 11-15: Moderate sleepiness
> 16-20: Severe sleepiness
> 21-24: Excessive sleepiness

> The patient's Epworth Sleepiness Scale is 16.

fracture classifications

See orthopedics

French scale

Sizing system for catheters, sounds, and other tubular instruments. Each unit is approximately 0.33 mm in diameter.

Express in arabic numerals.

Precede by # or *No.* if the word "number" is dictated.

Do not lowercase *French*.

> 5-French catheter
> #5-French catheter
> catheter, size 5 French

Keep in mind that *French* is linked to diameter size and is not the eponymic name of an instrument. Thus, it is a 15-French catheter, not a French catheter, size 15.

Glasgow coma scale

Describes level of consciousness of patients with head injuries by testing the patient's ability to respond to verbal, motor, and sensory stimulation.

Each parameter is scored on a scale of 1 through 5, then totals are added together to indicate level of consciousness. (Glasgow refers to Glasgow, Scotland.)

score	level of consciousness
14 or 15	normal
7 or less	coma
3 or less	brain death

global assessment of functioning (GAF) scale

A scale used by mental health professionals to assess an individual's overall psychological functioning. Typically reported in a psychiatric diagnosis as axis V.

Use arabic numerals 0 (inadequate information) through 100 (superior functioning in a wide range of activities).

> Axis V   GAF = 60   Flat affect.

See diagnosis *for a more complete discussion of psychiatric diagnoses.*

C

global assessment of relational functioning (GARF) scale

This scale is used by mental health professionals to measure an overall functioning of a family or other ongoing relationship. Use arabic numerals from 0 (inadequate information) to 100 (relational unit functioning satisfactorily from self-report of participants and from perspectives of observers).

GVHD grading system

Grading system for **graft-versus-host d**isease.

Use arabic numerals 1 (mild) through 4 (severe), placed on the line directly after the abbreviation (no space). May also be expressed as clinical grade 1 through 4.

> GVHD1 *or* GVHD clinical grade 1
> GVHD2 *or* GVHD clinical grade 2
> GVHD3 *or* GVHD clinical grade 3
> GVHD4 *or* GVHD clinical grade 4

Harvard criteria for brain death

In addition to body temperature equal to or higher than 32°C and the absence of central nervous system depressants, all of the following criteria must be met in order to establish brain death.

- unreceptivity and unresponsiveness

- no movement or breathing

- no reflexes

- flat electroencephalogram (confirmatory)

Hunt and Hess neurological classification

Classifies prognosis of patients with hemorrhage.

Write out and lowercase *grade*; do not abbreviate.

Use arabic numerals 1 through 4.

grade 3

Kurtzke disability score
Two-part scoring system to evaluate patients with multiple sclerosis.

Part one evaluates functional systems (pyramidal, cerebellar, brain stem, sensory, bowel and bladder, visual, mental, and other).

Part two is a disability status scale from 0 to 10.

Use arabic numerals.

magnitude scale
Measures earthquake magnitude. A one-unit increase on the scale equals a tenfold increase in ground motion.

Express with arabic numerals and decimal point.

She was injured in an earthquake measuring 6.6 magnitude.

Mallampati-Samsoon classification of airway
With the patient seated upright, mouth opened as wide as possible and tongue protruding, the anesthesiologist examines the airway—soft palate, tonsillar fauces, tonsillar pillars, and uvula—to evaluate the ease or difficulty of intubation: class I (easy intubation) through class IV (nearly impossible intubation).

Lowercase *class* and use roman numerals.

NYHA classification of cardiac failure

Use roman numerals I (asymptomatic) through IV (severe cardiac failure).

See cardiology

Outerbridge scale

Assesses damage in chondromalacia patellae.

Lowercase *grade*.

Use arabic numerals 1 (minimal) through 4 (excessive).

> Diagnosis: Chondromalacia patellae, grade 3.

physical status classification

A classification developed by the American Society of Anesthesiologists to classify a patient's risk of complications from surgery.

Lowercase *class* and use arabic numerals (1 through 5). The capital letter *E* is added to indicate an emergency operation.

> class 1E

Rancho Los Amigos cognitive function scale

Neurologic assessment tool. Levels I through VIII are written with roman numerals.

I	no response
II	generalized response to stimulation
III	localized response to stimuli
IV	confused and agitated behavior
V	confused with inappropriate behavior (nonagitated)
VI	confused but appropriate behavior

| VII | automatic and appropriate behavior |
| VIII | purposeful and appropriate behavior |

social and occupational functioning assessment scale (SOFAS)

The SOFAS is an instrument used by mental health professionals to assess an individual's social and occupational functioning only (**See** *also* global assessment of functioning (GAF) scale *above*).

Use arabic numerals from 0 (inadequate information) through 100 (superior functioning in a wide range of activities).

TIMI system

See cardiology terminology

trauma score

Scoring system that measures systolic blood pressure, respiratory rate and expansion, capillary refill, eye opening, and verbal and motor responses on a scale of 2 through 16. Score predicts injury severity and probability of survival.

Use arabic numerals.

clause

A clause is a group of words with a subject and verb. A clause may be a complete sentence or part of one.

independent clause

Also known as *main clause* or *principal clause*, an independent clause can stand alone as a sentence.

The patient came into the emergency room.

Use a comma to separate independent clauses joined by a conjunction (*and, but, for, or, nor, yet,* or *so*). The comma is optional if the main clauses are short and their meanings will not be confused.

> The platysma was then divided in the direction of its fibers, and blunt dissection was performed so that the prevertebral space was entered.
> A consultation was obtained, and liver function studies were done.
> A consultation was obtained and surgery was scheduled.

Use a semicolon instead of a comma when one or both of the independent clauses have internal commas, or when the second clause is closely linked to the first without a conjunction.

> The uterus, which was quite friable, was incised in its lower segment; flaps were created.
> He had numerous complaints; several were inconsistent with one another. *(two closely linked independent clauses joined by a semicolon)*

A colon may be used instead of a semicolon to separate two independent clauses when the second one explains or expands upon the first. **See** dependent clause *below*.

> He had numerous complaints: several were inconsistent with one another.

dependent clause
One that is subordinate to or depends on the independent clause; also known as a *subordinate clause*. It has a subject and a verb, but it cannot stand alone; hence its name. It may be introduced by such terms as *who, whom, that, which, when, after, although, before, if, whether.* **See** independent clause *above*.

In the following example, the dependent clause is in italics.

> The gallbladder, *although it was inflamed,* was without stones.

dependent essential clause

Dependent clause that cannot be eliminated without changing the meaning of the sentence; also known as a *restrictive clause.*

Use *who* or *whom* to introduce an essential clause referring to a human being or to an animal with a name.

Use *that* to introduce an essential clause referring to an inanimate object or to an animal without a name.

Exception: When *that* as a conjunction is used elsewhere in the same sentence, use *which*, not *that*, to introduce an *essential clause.*

> It was felt that the procedure which would be curative carried too great a risk.

Do not use commas to set off dependent essential clauses. *See* dependent nonessential clause *below.*

In the following sentences, the essential clauses are in italics.

> When the patient came into the emergency room she was treated for tachycardia *that had resisted conversion in her physician's office.*
> She had 2 large wounds *that were bleeding profusely* and several small bleeders.

dependent nonessential clause

Dependent clause that can be eliminated without changing the meaning of the sentence; also known as *nonrestrictive clause.*

Use commas to set off nonessential subordinate clauses or nonessential participial phrases.

Use *who* or *whom* to introduce a nonessential clause referring to a human being or an animal with a name. Use *which* to introduce a nonessential

HINT: *Which* is usually preceded by a comma; *that* is not.

clause referring to an inanimate object or to an animal without a name. *See* dependent essential clause *above*.

> The patient, *who was referred by her family physician,* came into the emergency room.
>
> The patient's parents, *who had been summoned from Europe,* were consulted about his past history.
>
> The incision, *which ran from the umbilicus to the symphysis pubis,* was closed in layers.
>
> The operation, *which began at 7 a.m.,* took 17 hours.

coordinate clause

One that is the same type as another (main to main, dependent to dependent). The following sentence has two main coordinate clauses separated by a comma and *and*.

> The patient came into the emergency room, and she was treated for tachycardia.

main clause

See independent clause *above*.

nonrestrictive clause

See dependent nonessential clause *above*.

principal clause

See independent clause *above*.

restrictive clause

See dependent essential clause *above*.

subordinate clause

See dependent clause *above*.

clipped sentences

See sentences

clock referents

When an anatomic position is described in terms of clockface orientation as seen by the viewer, use *o'clock* unless the position is subdivided.

The incision was made at the 3 o'clock position.

D: The cyst was found at the 2:30 o'clock position.
T: The cyst was found at the 2:30 position.

clotting factors

Lowercase *factor*. Use roman numerals.

factor I	fibrinogen
factor II	prothrombin
factor III	thromboplastin
factor IV	calcium ions
factor V	proaccelerin
factor VI	(none currently designated)
factor VII	proconvertin
factor VIII	antihemophilic factor
factor IX	Christmas factor
factor X	Stuart factor
factor XI	plasma thromboplastin antecedent
factor XII	glass factor
factor XIII	fibrin-stabilizing factor

C

platelet factors

Use arabic numerals for platelet factors (abbreviation: *PF*).

platelet factor 3
PF 3 *(Note: Space between* PF *and the numeral.)*

activated form

Add a lowercase *a* to designate a factor's activated form.

factor Xa

von Willebrand (factor VIII)

Newer terms for factor VIII (also known as *von Willebrand factor*) are preferred, but older terms continue to be used. Transcribe the dictated form, expressing it appropriately.

old term	*newer term*
factor VIII:C	factor VIII
factor VIII:CAg	factor VIII:Ag
von Willebrand factor	vWF
factor VIII:RAg	vWF:Ag
VIII:RCoF	ristocetin cofactor

cm

Abbreviation for *centimeter*.

Do not use periods. Do not add *s* for plural. Do not use fractions with metric units of measure. Space between the numeral and the abbreviation.

5 cm
5.5 cm *not* 5-1/2 cm

C

code, coding

A number or a number-letter combination assigned to a diagnosis or procedure or other healthcare terminology. Used for classification, reimbursement, research, and statistical purposes.

Coding systems include

abbreviation	coding system	publisher
IC	*The International Statistical Classification of Diseases and Related Health Problems*	Word Health Organization
CPT	*Current Procedural Terminology*	American Medical Association
HCPCS	Health Care Procedure Coding System	Centers for Medicare and Medicaid Services
SNOMED	Systematized Nomenclature of Medicine	American College of Pathologists
DSM	*Diagnostic and Statistical Manual of Mental Disorders*	American Psychiatric Association

coined terms

See language to avoid

college, College

Capitalize this term only when it is part of a proper name.

Modesto Junior College

college bookstore

American College of Obstetricians and Gynecologists

colons

The primary function of a colon as a punctuation mark is to introduce what follows: a list, series, or enumeration; an example; and sometimes a quotation (instead of a comma). Use either a single character space or two spaces following a colon, depending on your department or company policy for spacing at the end of a sentence; be consistent.

> She said: "I have never gotten along with my mother, and I no longer try."
>
> *or* She said, "I have never gotten along with my mother, and I no longer try."

Do not use a colon to introduce words that fit properly into the grammatical structure of the sentence without the colon, for example, after a verb, between a preposition and its object, or after *because*.

> The patient is on Glucophage, furosemide, and Vasotec. (*no colon after* on)
>
> He came to the emergency room because he was experiencing fever and chills of several hours' duration. (*no colon after* because)

> HEENT: PERRLA, EOMI.
>
> *or* HEENT shows PERRLA, EOMI.
>
> *not* HEENT shows: PERRLA, EOMI.

Capitalize the word following the colon if it is normally capitalized, if it follows a section or subsection heading, or if the list or series that follows the colon includes one or more complete sentences. Lowercase the first letter of each item in a series following a colon when the items are separated by commas.

> The patient is on the following medications: Theo-Dur, prednisone, Bronkometer.
>
> ABDOMEN: Benign.

> Pelvic examination revealed the following: Moderately atrophic vulva. Markedly atrophic vaginal mucosa.
>
> *or* Pelvic examination revealed the following: moderately atrophic vulva, markedly atrophic vaginal mucosa.
>
> *or* Pelvic examination revealed moderately atrophic vulva, markedly atrophic vaginal mucosa. (*no colon required*)

A colon may be used instead of a semicolon to separate two main clauses when the second one explains or expands upon the first.

> He had numerous complaints; several were inconsistent with one another.
>
> *or* He had numerous complaints: several were inconsistent with one another.

The colon is also used in numeric expressions of equator readings, ratios, and time.

A colon may introduce a series or follow a heading or subheading, and it may replace a dash in some instances.

commas

Use a comma to indicate a break in thought, to set off material, and to introduce a new but connected thought.

Sometimes a comma **must** be used; sometimes it **must not** be used; sometimes its use is **optional**. Use commas when the rules require them and when they enhance clarity, improve readability, or diminish confusion or misunderstanding. Avoid their overuse.

The rules for comma usage appear under a variety of topics throughout this book. Several are mentioned here as well.

adjectives

Use commas to separate two or more adjectives if each modifies the noun alone.

> Physical exam reveals a *pleasant, cooperative, slender* lady in no acute distress.

HINT: If you can replace the comma between adjectives with *and*, the comma is necessary.

Use commas to set off an adjective or adjectival phrase directly following the noun it modifies.

> He has degenerative arthritis, left knee, with increasing inability to cope.

appositives
Use commas before and after nonessential (or parenthetical) appositives.

> The surgeons, Dr. Jones and Dr. Smith, reported that the procedure was a success.

conjunctions
clauses
Use a comma to separate independent clauses joined by a conjunction.

> A consultation was obtained, and liver function studies were done.

coordinating conjunctions
Place a comma before a coordinating conjunction.

> He was seen in the emergency room, but he was not admitted.

subordinating conjunctions
Place a comma before a subordinating conjunction in most cases.

> He was in great pain, yet he refused treatment.

however
Place a semicolon before and a comma after *however* when it is used as a conjunctive adverb, connecting two complete, closely related thoughts in a single sentence.

> He is improved; however, he cannot be released.

Place a comma after *however* when it serves as a bridge between two sentences.

> The patient was released from care. However, his wife called to say his condition had worsened again.

When *however* occurs in the second sentence and is not the first word, it is called an interruptive and requires a comma before and after it (unless it appears at the end of the sentence).

> D&T: He is improved. He cannot, however, be released.
> D&T: He is improved. He cannot be released, however.

dates

When the month, day, and year are given in this sequence, set off the year by commas.

> She was admitted on December 14, 2001, and discharged on January 4, 2002.

genetics

Place a comma (without spacing) between the chromosome number and the sex chromosome. Use a virgule to indicate more than one karyotype in an individual.

> The normal human karyotypes are 46,XX (female) and 46,XY (male).

geographic names

In text, use a comma before and after the state name preceded by a city name, or a country name preceded by a state or city name.

> The patient moved to Modesto, California, 15 years ago.

> The patient returned from a business trip to Paris, France, the week prior to admission.

lists and series

Lists can take many forms. One style is a run-on (horizontal, narrative) list that uses commas or semicolons between items in the list.

> He was sent home on Biaxin 500 mg b.i.d., Atrovent inhaler 2 puffs q.i.d., and Altace 5 mg daily.
>
> Her past history includes (1) diabetes mellitus, (2) cholecystitis, (3) hiatal hernia.

Using a final comma before the conjunction preceding the last item in a series is optional unless its presence or absence changes the meaning.

> Ears, nose, and throat are normal. *(final comma optional)*
>
> No dysphagia, hoarseness, or enlargement of the thyroid gland. *(final comma required)*
>
> The results showed blood sugar 46%, creatinine and BUN normal. (*no comma after* creatinine)

parenthetical expressions

Set off parenthetical expressions by commas.

> A great deal of swelling was present, more so on the left than on the right.

Use a comma before and after Latin abbreviations (and their translations), such as *etc., i.e., e.g., et al., viz.,* when they are used as parenthetical expressions within a sentence.

> Her symptoms come on with exertion, for example, when climbing stairs or running.

> Her symptoms come on with exertion, e.g., when climbing stairs or running.

quotation marks

Always place the comma following a quotation inside the closing quotation mark.

The patient stated that "the itching is driving me crazy," and she scratched her arms throughout our meeting.

titles

Lowercase job titles that are set off from a name by commas.

The pathology department secretary, John Smith, called us with the preliminary report.

units of measure

Do not use a comma or other punctuation between units of the same dimension.

The infant weighed 5 pounds 3 ounces.

complement factors

Factors involved in antigen-antibody reactions and inflammation.

Immediately follow a capital *C, B, P,* or *D* with an arabic numeral on the line.

C1
C7

Add a lowercase letter (usually *a* or *b*) for fragments of complement components.

C5a
Bb

compound modifiers

A compound modifier consists of two or more words that act as a unit modifying a noun or pronoun. The use of hyphens to join these words varies depending on the type of compound modifier, as indicated below.

Some compound modifiers are so commonly used together, or are so clear, that they are automatically read as a unit and do not need to be joined with hyphens.

> dark brown lesion
> deep tendon reflexes
> 1st trimester bleeding
> jugular venous distention
> left lower quadrant
> low back pain
> ST-T wave abnormality
> 3rd degree burn

adjective ending in -ly

Use a hyphen in a compound modifier beginning with an adjective that ends in *-ly*. (This requires distinguishing between adjectives ending in *-ly* and adverbs ending in *-ly*.) Do not use a hyphen with compound modifiers containing an adverb ending in *-ly*.

> scholarly-looking patient
> *but* quickly paced steps

adjective-noun compound

Use a hyphen in an adjective-noun compound that precedes and modifies another noun. *See* noun-adjective compound *below*.

> second-floor office
> *but* The office is on the second floor.

adjective with preposition

Use hyphens in most compound adjectives that contain a preposition.

> finger-to-nose test

adjective with participle

Use a hyphen to join an adjective to a participle, whether the compound precedes or follows the noun.

> good-natured, soft-spoken patient
> The patient is good-natured and soft-spoken.

adverb with participle or adjective

Use a hyphen to form a compound modifier made up of an adverb coupled with a participle or adjective when they precede the noun they modify but not when they follow it.

> well-developed and well-nourished woman
> *but* The patient was well developed and well nourished.

> fast-acting medication
> *but* The medication is fast acting.

adverb ending in -ly

Do not use a hyphen in a compound modifier to link an adverb ending in -*ly* with a participle or adjective.

> recently completed workup
> moderately acute pain
> financially stable investment

adverb preceding a compound modifier

Do not use a hyphen in a compound modifier preceded by an adverb.

> somewhat well nourished patient

very

Drop the hyphen in a compound modifier with a participle or adjective when it is preceded by the adverb *very*.

very well developed patient

disease-entity modifiers

Do not use hyphens with most disease-entity modifiers even when they precede the noun. Check appropriate medical references for guidance.

cervical disk disease

oat cell carcinoma

pelvic inflammatory disease

sickle cell disease

urinary tract infection

but insulin-dependent diabetes mellitus *and* non-insulin-dependent diabetes mellitus

eponyms

Use a hyphen to join two or more eponymic names used as multiple-word modifiers of diseases, operations, procedures, instruments, etc.

Do not use a hyphen if the multiple-word, eponymic name refers to a single person.

Use appropriate medical references to differentiate.

Osgood-Schlatter disease *(named for US orthopedic surgeon Robert B. Osgood and Swiss surgeon Carl Schlatter)*

Chevalier Jackson forceps *(named for Chevalier Jackson, US pioneer in bronchoesophagology)*

equal, complementary, or contrasting adjectives

Use a hyphen to join two adjectives that are equal, complementary, or contrasting when they precede or follow the noun they modify.

> anterior-posterior infarction
>
> physician-patient confidentiality issues
>
> His eyes are blue-green.

foreign expressions

Do not hyphenate foreign expressions used in compound adjectives, even when they precede the noun they modify (unless they are always hyphenated).

> in vitro experiments
>
> carcinoma in situ
>
> cul-de-sac *(always hyphenated)*
>
> ex officio member

high- and low-

Use a hyphen in most *high-* and *low-* compound adjectives.

> high-density mass
>
> low-frequency waves
>
> high-power field

noun-adjective compound

Use a hyphen to join some noun-adjective compounds (but not all). Check appropriate references (dictionaries and grammar books).

When a hyphen is appropriate, use it whether the noun-adjective compound precedes or follows the noun it is modifying.

> It is a medication-resistant condition.
>
> *or* The condition was medication-resistant.

This is a symptom-free patient.
or The patient was symptom-free.

Stool is heme-negative.

noun with participle

Use a hyphen to join a noun and a participle to form a compound modifier whether it comes before or after a noun.

bone-biting forceps
She was panic-stricken.
mucus-coated throat (*the throat was coated with* mucus, *not* mucous)
callus-forming lesion (*the lesion was forming* callus, *not* callous)

numerals with words

Use a hyphen between a number and a word forming a compound modifier preceding a noun.

3-week history
5 x 3 x 2-cm mass
2-year 5-month-old child
8-pound 5-ounce baby girl

proper nouns as adjective

Do not use hyphens in proper nouns even when they serve as a modifier preceding a noun.

John F. Kennedy High School
New Mexico residents

Do not use hyphens in combinations of proper noun and common noun serving as a modifier.

> Tylenol capsule administration

series of hyphenated compound modifiers

Use a suspensive hyphen after each incomplete modifier when there is a series of hyphenated compound modifiers with a common last word that is expressed only after the final modifier in the series.

> 10- to 12-year history
> 3- to 4-cm lesion
> full- and split-thickness grafts

If one or more of the incomplete modifiers is not hyphenated, repeat the base with each, hyphenating or not, as appropriate.

> preoperative and postoperative diagnoses (*not* pre- and postoperative diagnoses)

to clarify or to avoid confusion

Use a hyphen to clarify meaning and to avoid confusion, absurdity, or ambiguity in compound modifiers. The hyphen may not be necessary if the meaning is made clear by the surrounding context.

> large-bowel obstruction (*obstruction of the large bowel,* not *a large obstruction of the bowel*)

hyphenated compound modifiers

Use a hyphen or en dash to join hyphenated compound modifiers or a hyphenated compound modifier with a one-word modifier.

> non-disease-entity modifier
> *or* non–disease-entity modifier

C

Use a hyphen or en dash to join two unhyphenated compound modifiers.

> the North Carolina-South Carolina border
> *or* the North Carolina–South Carolina border

Use a hyphen or en dash to join an unhyphenated compound modifier with a hyphenated one.

> beta-receptor-mediated response (*or* ß-receptor-mediated response)
> *or* beta-receptor–mediated response (*or* ß-receptor–mediated response)

Use a hyphen or en dash to join an unhyphenated compound modifier with a one-word modifier.

> vitamin D-deficiency rickets
> *or* vitamin D–deficiency rickets

compound words

Compound words may be written as one or multiple words; check dictionaries, grammar books, and other appropriate references.

hyphens

Hyphens are always used in some compound words, sometimes used in others, and never used in still others. Check dictionaries and other appropriate references for guidance.

> attorney at law
> beta-blocker
> chief of staff
> father-in-law
> half-life

near-syncope

vice president

Use a hyphen to join two nouns that are equal, complementary, or contrasting.

blood-brain barrier

fracture-dislocation

Do not hyphenate proper nouns of more than one word, even when they serve as a modifier preceding a noun.

South Dakota residents

Do not use a hyphen in a combination of proper noun and common noun.

Tylenol capsule administration

Use a hyphen with all compound nouns containing *ex-* when *ex-* means former and precedes a noun that can stand on its own.

ex-wife

ex-president

Use a hyphen in compound verbs unless one of the terms is a preposition.

single-space

but follow up

compound words

HINT: To test whether the correct form is one word or two, try changing the tense or number. If one or more letters must be added, the correct form is two words.

We will follow up.

tense change >>

We followed up.

(*Followedup* is not a word, so *followed up* must be two words.)

We follow up.

number change >>

He follows up.

(*Followsup* is not a word, so *follows up* must be two words.)

Sometimes hyphenated compound words become so well established that the hyphen is dropped and the words are joined together without a hyphen. When such a word can be used as either a noun, adjective, or verb, the noun and adjective forms are joined without a hyphen, but the verb form remains two separate words if one of them is a preposition.

noun, adjective	*verb*
checkup	check up
followup	follow up
workup	work up
followthrough	follow through

The patient was lost to followup. *(noun)*
Followup exam will be in 3 weeks. *(adjective)*
I will follow up the patient in 3 weeks. *(verb)*

Some terms consisting of a word followed by a single letter or symbol are hyphenated; others are not. Check appropriate references for guidance.

> type 1 diabetes
> vitamin D
> Dukes A carcinoma

Some terms with a single letter or symbol followed by a word are hyphenated, others are not. Check appropriate references for guidance, and consider the use of hyphens in such terms as optional if you are unable to document. Even if such terms are unhyphenated in their noun form, they should be hyphenated in their adjective form.

> B-complex vitamins
> T wave
> T-wave abnormality
> x-rays
> x-ray results

When a Greek letter is part of the name, use a hyphen after the symbol but not after the spelled-out form.

> ß-carotene *but* beta carotene

plurals

For those written as a single word, form the plural by adding *s*.

> fingerbreadths
> tablespoonfuls
> workups

For those formed by a noun and modifier(s), form the plural by making the noun plural.

> sisters-in-law

For plural compound nouns containing a possessive, make the second noun plural.

> associate's degrees
> driver's licenses

For some compound nouns, the plural is formed irregularly.

> forget-me-nots

possessive forms

Use *'s* after the last word in a hyphenated compound term.

> daughter-in-law's inquiry

confidentiality

Patients have a legal and ethical right to the reasonable expectation that their private information will not be disclosed except for the purposes for which it was provided (such as receiving healthcare services). Medical transcriptionists share with other healthcare personnel the responsibility to respect the confidentiality of medical records. Federal and state laws govern the extent of confidentiality required and the exceptions under which disclosure can be made.

Confidentiality is sometimes confused with two related but different concepts: privacy and privilege. Privacy means an individual's right to be left alone and/or to decide what to share with others. Privacy may, for example, affect whether gratuitous, irrelevant, and personal information is even included in a record. Privilege means the legal protection against being forced to violate confidentiality in a legal proceeding, such as by disclosing confidential records.

HIPAA privacy rule

The Health Insurance Portability and Accountability Act of 1996 (HIPAA) includes regulations related to the privacy of health information. The HIPAA privacy rule requires healthcare providers and others who maintain health information to put in place measures to guard the privacy and confidentiality of patient information. Before HIPAA, patient privacy was only sporadically protected by various laws—never so dramatically as it is by the HIPAA statute and its accompanying regulations. The text of the rule, published in the Federal Register on December 28, 2000, can be found on the Administrative Simplification website of the US Department of Health and Human Services: http://aspe.hhs.gov/admnsimp.

Some states may have more stringent privacy requirements than those contained in the HIPAA privacy rule. It behooves every medical transcription business owner to understand the applicable state laws and make a determination as to which is more stringent, and the business owner should seek the advice of an attorney in this regard.

protecting patient information

The HIPAA privacy rule regulates the use and disclosure of specifically identifiable health information regarding the physical or mental health or condition of an individual. The rule applies **directly** to those entities that typically generate individually identifiable patient health information and therefore have primary responsibility for maintaining the privacy and confidentiality of such information. As a general matter, a so-called "covered entity" may use or disclose protected health information only with an individual's written consent or authorization. However, health information can be disclosed without consent or authorization for certain purposes, such as research and public health, if specified conditions are met. Covered entities also must comply with a host of administrative requirements intended to protect patient privacy.

The privacy rule also applies **indirectly** to business associates of covered entities. Medical transcriptionists who contract directly with healthcare providers fall into this category. The privacy rule requires covered entities to enter into a written agreement with each business associate—known as a business associate agreement. Significantly, the business associate may not use or disclose the protected health information other than as permitted or required by the business associate agreement or as required by law. Subcontractors must agree to essentially the same conditions and restrictions as business associates with respect to the use and disclosure of protected health information.

Within the body of the medical report, care should be taken to avoid mentioning personally identifying information. For example, it is common practice for a medical transcriptionist to replace the dictated patient's name with simply "the patient" or perhaps, "the above-named patient." What follows is a list of identifiers that are best avoided in medical reports, whether in reference to a patient or to a patient's relatives, employers, or household members.

> name
> address
> dates (e.g., date of birth, admission and discharge dates)
> telephone and fax numbers
> email addresses
> Social Security numbers

medical record numbers

health plan beneficiary numbers

account numbers

certificate/license numbers

vehicle identifiers, including license plate numbers

device identifiers and serial numbers

Web Universal Resource Locators (URL)

Internet protocol (IP) address numbers

biometric identifiers (e.g., finger and voice prints)

full-face photographic images and any comparable images

any other unique identifying number, characteristic, or code

Note: The HIPAA privacy rule makes clear provisions for "de-identifying" a record so that it is no longer considered protected health information. While the above list of identifiers is similar to the list found in the privacy rule, if your intention is to actually de-identify the record you will need to refer to the rule itself—as well as legal counsel—for specific guidelines.

retention of records

For the medical transcriptionist, discussions about retaining healthcare records generally apply to patient logs, dictated tapes or digital voice files, and transcribed reports (whether print or electronic). AAMT recommends that independent MTs and MT businesses retain such information only as long as is absolutely necessary to conduct business, that is, no longer than necessary for verification, distribution, and billing purposes. This opinion is shared by the authors of ASTM's *E1902, Standard Guide for Management of the Confidentiality and Security of Dictation, Transcription, and Transcribed Health Records.*

See security

conjunctions

Words that join words, phrases, or clauses, thereby indicating their relationship.

Examples: *and, but, for, however, or, nor, yet, so.*

conjunctive adverbs

Conjunctive adverbs connect two independent clauses. They include *consequently, finally, furthermore, however, moreover, nevertheless, similarly, subsequently, then, therefore, thus*. Precede a conjunctive adverb by a semicolon (sometimes a period), and usually follow it by a comma.

> She reported feeling better; however, her fever still spiked in the evenings.
> He was admitted through the emergency room; then he was taken to surgery.

coordinating conjunctions

Coordinating conjunctions *(and, but, or, nor, for)* join separate main clauses. They are usually preceded by a comma, sometimes by a semicolon, occasionally a colon.

> He was seen in the emergency room, but he was not admitted.

Do not use a comma before a coordinating conjunction that is followed by a second verb without a new subject.

> The patient tolerated the procedure well and left the department in stable condition.
> The gallbladder was inflamed but without stones.

subordinating conjunctions

Subordinating conjunctions *(while, where, since, after, yet, so)* connect two unequal parts, e.g., dependent and independent clauses. Precede a subordinating conjunction by a comma in most cases.

> He was in great pain, yet he refused treatment.

correlative conjunctions

Terms or phrases used in pairs, e.g., *either...or, neither...nor,* and *not only...but also*.

C

With an *either...or* or *neither...nor* construction, match the number of the verb with the number of the nearest subject.

> Neither the sister nor the brothers exhibit similar symptoms.
> Neither the brothers nor the sister exhibits similar symptoms.

If the subjects before and after *or* or *nor* are both singular, use a singular verb; if both subjects are plural, use a plural verb.

> Neither the sister nor the brother exhibits similar symptoms.
> Neither the sisters nor the brothers exhibit similar symptoms.

not only...but also

Check usage for parallelism; recast as necessary.

If *also* is omitted, insert it or some other word(s) for balance.

> D: He could not only be stubborn but offensive.
> T: He could be not only stubborn but also offensive.
> *or* He could be not only stubborn but offensive as well.

consensus

Note spelling. The term, derived from *consent* (not *census*), means an agreement or decision reached by a group as a whole (they consent).

The phrase *consensus of opinion* is redundant; *consensus* is adequate.

consultation report

A consultation includes examination, review, and assessment of a patient by a healthcare provider other than the attending physician. The report generated is called a consultation report. The consulting specialist directs the report to the physician requesting the consultation, usually the attending physician. Content usually includes patient examination, review, and assessment. It may be prepared in letter or report format.

See Appendix A: Sample Reports

continuation pages
See formats

contractions

Words with missing letters or numbers denoted by apostrophes.

Avoid contractions except in direct quotations.

dictated	*transcribed*
can't	cannot
I'd	I would *or* I had
he's	he is *or* he has
it's	it is *or* it has

Where possible, extend abbreviations that contain contractions.

D: The patient OD'd on...
T: The patient overdosed on...

D: Stool was guaiac'd.
T: Guaiac test was done on the stool.

When using contractions, take care to place the apostrophe correctly.

The mother reported, "He's been hysterical."

copy designation
See correspondence

correspondence
Patient reports often are written in the form of a letter to a referring or consulting physician. The fonts, styles, and margins chosen for use in letters may differ from those used in other medical reports; each department (or client) will develop its own policies. The following types of correspondence are demonstrated in Appendix A: Sample Reports.

letter formats and styles
Margins for letters are often determined by the letterhead used. It is not uncommon in long letters that additional pages conform to different margins, depending on the paper used. Be sure to review the letterhead and continuation sheets (the paper used for additional pages after the first letterhead page) to adjust the left, right, top, and bottom margins as needed.

In the full block format (*See* Appendix A: Sample Reports *for examples*), all text begins flush with the left margin. This includes the date, address, reference line, salutation, the body of the letter with double spacing for each new paragraph, the complimentary close, and signature line. Tabs are not used as all paragraphs are flush left.

In the modified block format, the date, complimentary close, and signature line are placed just to the right of the middle of the page. An acceptable variation of the modified block allows each new paragraph within the text of the body of the letter to be double spaced and indented five spaces or about ¼ inch.

address
Use commas to separate the parts of an address in narrative form. Exception: Do not place a comma before the ZIP code.

The patient's address is 139 Main Street, Ourtown, CA 90299.

Always use figures (including 1) to refer to house numbers. Do not use commas.

> 1 Eighth Avenue
> 1408 51st Street
> 101st Street
> 14084 Elm Avenue

Use *No.* or *#* before an apartment, suite, or room number but not before a house number.

> 1400 Magnolia Avenue, Apt. #148

salutation

Greeting line in letters *(Dear...).* Use courtesy titles *(Dr., Ms, etc.),* followed by a colon or a comma, according to letter style and format you use.

Note: While salutation lines continue to be the preferred and common practice, it is acceptable to drop them in form letters or in those instances when the appropriate courtesy title is not known, for example, when you cannot determine whether the person is male or female. *To Whom It May Concern* is another alternative in that instance, but it appears to be losing favor.

copy designation

Notation of those to whom copies of a report or letter are to be distributed.

A carbon copy is increasingly known as a *courtesy copy.* Abbreviated *cc.*

A blind copy designation is noted only on the file copy and on the copy to whom it is sent; other recipients' copies do not indicate the blind copy (thus its name). Abbreviated *bc* or *bcc.*

Place copy designations flush left and two line spaces below the end of the report.

bc	blind copy
bcc	blind courtesy copy
c	copy
cc	courtesy copy, carbon copy
pc	photocopy

envelope preparation

The US Postal Service offers the following guidelines on their website at www.usps.com.

Automated mail processing machines read addresses on mailpieces from the bottom up and will first look for a city, state, and ZIP code. Then the machines look for a delivery address. If the machines can't find either line, then your mailpiece could be delayed or misrouted. Any information below the delivery address line (a logo, a slogan, or an attention line) could confuse the machines and misdirect your mail.

Name or attention line	JANE L MILLER
Company	MILLER ASSOCIATES
Suite or apartment number	[STE 2006]
Delivery address	1960 W CHELSEA AVE STE 2006
City, state, ZIP code	ALLENTOWN PA 18104

- Always put the recipient's address and the postage on the same side of your mailpiece.
- On a letter, the address should be parallel to the longest side.
- Use all capital letters.
- No punctuation.
- At least 10-point font.
- One space between city and state.

- Simple fonts and regular (plain) type.
- Left justified.
- Black type on white or light paper.
- No reverse type styles (white printing on a black background).
- If your address appears inside a window, make sure there is at least 1/8-inch clearance around the address. Sometimes parts of the address slip out of view behind the window and mail processing machines can't read the address.
- If you are using address labels, make sure you don't cut off any important information. Also make sure your labels are on straight. Mail processing machines have trouble reading crooked or slanted information.

email

Email has become an important communication medium.

security

When email is used for sending and receiving confidential patient information, whether voice or text files, reasonable precautions should be taken to ensure the protection of that information. Federal privacy and security regulations demand it, and state and local laws may also apply.

etiquette

Here are some etiquette essentials to help you use email efficiently and effectively.

- Keep your messages short and simple. This is not the place for a novel.
- Do not write your entire message in uppercase. It is equivalent to shouting, and it is not pleasant or easy to read. SEE WHAT I MEAN?
- Go easy on the abbreviations. Unless you can be sure the reader knows all of your abbreviations, the meaning of your message may be lost.
- Use blind cc when sending a mass message. Your recipients will appreciate your respect of their personal email addresses.

- Close your message with your name. Don't assume that the reader will recognize you by your email address.
- Don't send junk, jokes, or chain letters unless you know the reader wants them.
- Don't send unsolicited attachments. When you do send an attachment, explain in your message what the attachment is, and be sure to scan it for viruses before you send it.
- Include only relevant return text. After several exchanges, the email expands to enormous proportions if complete messages are included.
- Use the spellchecker. Misspelled words don't reflect well on the sender and can be annoying to the reader.
- Use a meaningful subject line. This will assist the reader when prioritizing the order of emails to read.
- Don't put anything in an email that you would not put on a postcard. Email is not ordinarily secure.

See confidentiality
security
Appendix A: Sample Reports

cranial nerves

Use arabic or roman numerals for cranial nerve designations. Be consistent. (Employer or client will often indicate preference.)

cranial nerve 12   cranial nerve XII
cranial nerves 2-12   cranial nerves II-XII

Ordinals should be expressed using arabic numerals or may be spelled out in full.

12th cranial nerve
or twelfth cranial nerve

English names are preferred to Latin, but transcribe Latin forms if they are dictated.

number	*English name*	*Latin name*
1 *or* I	olfactory	olfactorius
2 *or* II	optic	opticus
3 *or* III	oculomotor	oculomotorius
4 *or* IV	trochlear	trochlearis
5 *or* V	trigeminal	trigeminus
6 *or* VI	abducens	abducens
7 *or* VII	facial	facialis
8 *or* VIII	vestibulocochlear	vestibulocochlearis
9 *or* IX	glossopharyngeal	glossopharyngeus
10 *or* X	vagus	vagus
11 *or* XI	accessory	accessorius
12 *or* XII	hypoglossal	hypoglossus

credentials, professional

Designations, such as MD, CMT, RHIA, that identify the professional degrees, certifications, licensures, or registrations carried by an individual.

abbreviated forms

Use abbreviated forms after a full name (not just a surname).

Do not use periods in most such abbreviations; follow the preferred style for the designation.

Use commas to set off professional credentials when they follow the person's name.

Nora Brown, MD

C

capitalization

Capitalize abbreviated forms, but do not capitalize the extended form unless it follows a person's name.

> a CMT
> a certified medical transcriptionist
> James Morrison, CMT
> Jane Smith, Doctor of Medicine

with initials

Do not use credentials after initials, as in originator-transcriptionist initials at the end of a report.

> JD:DH *not* JDMD:DHCMT

false credentials

Do not place abbreviations that are not recognized designations for professional credentials or academic degrees after your (or anyone else's) name.

> Mary Frank
> *not* Mary Frank, MT
> *not* Mary Frank, MLS

multiple credentials

If the individual holds multiple professional credentials, present them in the order preferred by the individual, with a comma (not a virgule) and a space between them.

> Betsy Worker, CMT, RHIA
> *not* Betsy Worker, CMT/RHIA

salutations

Do not use credentials in salutations.

Dear Dr. Smith:

not Dear Dr. Smith, DPM:

See Appendix I: Professional Credentials and Academic Degrees

crepitance, crepitation, crepitus

Crepitus, *crepitation*, and *crepitance* are all synonymous.

The adjectival form is *crepitant* ("crepitants" is not a word).

Although *crepitance* is not found in dictionaries, its frequent usage has made it acceptable.

D

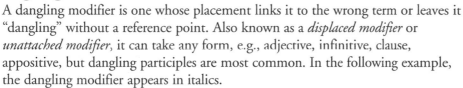

D

D as abbreviation for *dictated* is used throughout this text to indicate what was dictated and to contrast it with what should be transcribed *(T)*.

dangling modifiers

A dangling modifier is one whose placement links it to the wrong term or leaves it "dangling" without a reference point. Also known as a *displaced modifier* or *unattached modifier*, it can take any form, e.g., adjective, infinitive, clause, appositive, but dangling participles are most common. In the following example, the dangling modifier appears in italics.

> *Entering the abdomen through a Pfannenstiel incision,* the omentum was noted to be bound down by adhesions.

In many instances it is prudent to transcribe dangling modifiers as dictated, provided they do not confuse or amuse, because they have become so common throughout medical dictation, particularly in surgical reports. Certainly, to edit multiple dangling modifiers in a single report may raise objections from originators that their style has been tampered with, and doing so could also be unreasonably time-consuming. Nevertheless, be alert to dangling modifiers and change the more ludicrous among them.

Following is the edited version of the example given above.

> The abdomen was entered through a Pfannenstiel incision, and the omentum was noted to be bound down by adhesions.

Some dangling participles have been legitimized because they are so commonly used and familiar; these include *judging, considering, assuming, concerning, given, owing to*, and *provided*.

> Provided he follows instructions, he should heal rapidly.
> Considering his medical history, his condition is remarkable.

dashes

Dashes are not required in medical transcription, and alternatives are readily available. Even when dashes are acceptable, their use should be minimized, because their overuse creates visual clutter that makes reading difficult.

Form a dash either by using the specific key (or key combination) offered by your keyboard, or by using two hyphens.

When dashes are used, do not space before or after them.

Replace dashes by commas wherever doing so will not distort the meaning or confuse the reader.

abrupt change in continuity
Use a comma or dash to introduce an abrupt change in continuity.

> The patient agreed to return tomorrow, if he felt like it.
> *or* The patient agreed to return tomorrow—if he felt like it.
> *or* The patient agreed to return tomorrow--if he felt like it.

clauses
Use commas instead of dashes to set off clauses that do not have internal commas.

The patient, who had multiple complaints, demanded to be seen immediately.
preferred to
The patient—who had multiple complaints—demanded to be seen immediately.

missing letters or numbers

Use a dash to represent missing letters or numbers. Be sure to place a space after the dash or double hyphen representing the ending letters or numbers in a term.

The patient said, "What the h— did he think I would do?"
or "What the h-- did he think I would do?"

data, datum

Data, the plural form of *datum*, usually takes a plural verb, but its use as a collective noun taking a singular verb is becoming widely accepted. The singular form, *datum*, is seldom used.

The data were collected over a period of several years.
The data demonstrates conclusive evidence that...
The research data were checked, datum by datum.

date dictated, date transcribed

These dates should be recorded to monitor dictation and transcription patterns as well as to provide documentation of when the work (dictation or transcription) was done. Some dictation and transcription systems are specially designed to automatically record these dates.

Healthcare reports are, among other things, legal documents. As part of risk management, dictation and transcription dates should be entered accurately and should not be altered.

Capitalize *D* and *T* and follow each by a colon and appropriate date, using numerals separated by virgules or hyphens.

D

Some facilities prefer to use six-digit dates and others, eight-digit. All these styles are acceptable.

> D: 4/18/00
> T: 4/19/00

> D: 04-18-00
> T: 04-19-00

> D: 04/18/2000
> T: 04/19/2000

Note: ASTM's *E2184, Standard Specification for Healthcare Document Formats* calls for identification of the place of dictation as well.

See audit trails
formats
risk management

dates
punctuation
When the month, day, and year are given in this sequence, set off the year by commas. Do not use ordinals.

> She was admitted on December 14, 2001, and discharged on January 4, 2002.
> *not* ...January 4th, 2002 (4th *is an ordinal*)

Do not use commas when the month and year are given without the day, or when the military date sequence (day, month, year) is used.

> She was admitted in December 2001 and discharged in January 2002.
> She was admitted on 14 December 2001 and discharged on 4 January 2002.

Do not use punctuation after the year if the date stands alone, as in admission and discharge dates on reports.

> Admission date: April 4, 2000
> Discharge date: April 5, 2000

ordinals

Use ordinals when the day of the month precedes the month and is preceded by *the*; do not use commas. Do not use ordinals in month/day/year format.

> the 4th of April 2001 *not* April 4th, 2001

military style

When the military style is used, the day precedes the month. Use numerals; do not use commas. Write out or abbreviate the month (without periods) and use arabic figures for day and year.

> 4 April 2001
> 4 Apr 2001

in text

It is preferable to spell out dates used in the body of a report, writing out the name of the month and using four digits for the year.

> The patient was previously seen on April 4, 2001.

However, if dates are used repeatedly, as in a long history or hospital course, they may be expressed as numerals separated by virgules or hyphens as long as they are clearly understood.

> Electrolytes on April 24, 2001, revealed a sodium of 135, potassium 4.3, bicarbonate 25, chlorides 102. Repeated on 4/25 and again on 4/26, electrolytes remained within normal limits.

When only the month and day are dictated, and not the year, add the year only if you are certain what year is being referred to.

> D: The patient was last seen on April 4th.
>
> T: The patient was last seen on April 4, 2001. *(only if you're sure it's 2001)*

end of line

Divide dates at the end of a line of text between the day and the year. Avoid dividing between the month and the day.

> ....February 17,
> 2001
>
> *not*
>
> ....February
> 17, 2001

days of the week

Capitalize the names of the days of the week.

Do not abbreviate them except in tables, where three-letter abbreviations without periods may be used.

Sunday	Sun
Monday	Mon
Tuesday	Tue
Wednesday	Wed
Thursday	Thu
Friday	Fri
Saturday	Sat

When referring to a day in a report, use the day's name and the date. Avoid terms such as *last* Monday or *next* Wednesday. For dates in previous or subsequent years, specify the year.

deci-

Prefix meaning *one-tenth of a unit.*

To convert to basic unit, move decimal point one place to the left.

> 18.3 decigrams = 1.83 grams
> 2 deciliters = 0.2 liters
> decibels

decimals, decimal units

Use numerals to express decimal amounts.

Use the period as a decimal point or indicator.

metric measurements

Always use the decimal form with metric units of measure, even when they are dictated as a fraction.

> D: The mass was two and a half centimeters in diameter.
> T: The mass was 2.5 cm in diameter.

Exception: When the originator uses a fraction that cannot be exactly translated into decimals, transcribe as dictated.

> D: one third centimeter
> T: 1/3 cm

D

When whole numbers are dictated, do not add a decimal point and zero because doing so may cause them to be misread. It also indicates a degree of specificity that, if not dictated, was not intended by the originator. This is critical with drug doses because the addition of a decimal point and zero could lead to serious consequences if misread as ten times the amount ordered.

> 2 mg
> *not* 2.0 mg

When the decimal point and zero following a whole number are dictated to emphasize the preciseness of a measurement, e.g., of a pathology specimen or a laboratory value, transcribe them as dictated. Do not, however, insert the decimal point and zero if they are not dictated.

> D&T: The specimen measured 4.8 x 2.0 x 3.4 mm.
> *but*
> D&T: The specimen measured 4.8 x 2 x 3.4 mm.

For quantities less than 1, place a zero before the decimal point, except when the number could never equal 1 (e.g., in bullet calibers and in certain statistical expressions such as correlation coefficients and statistical probability).

> 0.75 mg
> .22-caliber rifle

Do not exceed two places following the decimal except in special circumstances, e.g., specific gravity values, or when a precise measurement is intended. ***See*** nonmetric forms of measure *below.*

> 0.624 K wire
> specific gravity 1.030

nonmetric forms of measure

Use the decimal form with nonmetric forms of measure when a precise measurement is intended and the fraction form would be both cumbersome and inexact. Two or more places may follow the decimal.

The 0.1816-inch screw was inserted.

degrees (°)

See the discussion on the use of degrees and the degree sign (°) under angles, classification systems (burn classifications), *and* temperature, temperature scales.

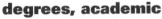

In handwritten chart notes the degree sign is often used to mean *hours* (as in "no urine output x8°") or *primary/secondary/tertiary* (1°, 2°, 3°), but the medical transcriptionist should translate these symbols to the appropriate terms.

degrees, academic

apostrophe

Use an apostrophe in degree designations such as *master's degree* or *bachelor's*.

capitalization

Do not capitalize generic forms of academic degrees.

bachelor's degree

master's

Use uppercase and lowercase abbreviations as appropriate.

Pharm D

PhD

DDS

Capitalize the expanded form only when it follows a person's name.

> Jane Smith, Licensed Clinical Social Worker

courtesy titles

When a courtesy title for an academic degree, e.g., *Dr.*, precedes a name, do not use the degree abbreviation after the name. Use one form or the other.

> Dr. Andrew Taylor Still
> *or* Andrew Taylor Still, DO
> *not* Dr. Andrew Taylor Still, DO

honorary degrees

Omit honorary degree designations.

> Jane Smith *not* Jane Smith, PhD (hon)

multiple degrees

Use the order preferred by the individual named, separating the degrees by commas. (In the case of publications, such as journals, the publication's editorial style prevails.)

In general, omit academic degrees below the master's level. If an individual has a doctoral degree, omit degrees at master's level or below, unless the master's degree represents a relevant but different or specialized field.

> John Smith, MD, MSW

Include specialized professional certifications if pertinent (CMT, CRNA, PA). Separate multiple degrees (and/or professional credentials) by commas.

> Jane Smith, RPh, PhD
> John Smith, CMT, RHIT

When an individual holds two doctorates, use either or both according to the individual's preference.

>   Jane Smith, MD, PhD

periods

While periods continue to be used in academic degrees, the preferred form is without them.

If periods are used, do not space within the abbreviation.

>   John Smith, BA *preferred to* John Smith, B.A. (*not* B. A.)
>   Jane Smith, PA-C

salutations and addresses

Use the courtesy title (with last name only) in salutations, the academic title (with full name) in addresses.

>   Dear Dr. Smith:
>   John Smith, MD *(in address)*

signature line

Always use the academic title, never the courtesy title, in signature lines.

>   Sincerely yours,

>   Jane Smith, MD (*not* Dr. Jane Smith)

D

with initials

Do not use degrees or credentials after initials, as in originator and transcriptionist initials at the end of a report.

> JD:DH
> *not* JDMD:DHCMT

with names

Place academic degrees after a full name (not just a surname). A comma is generally placed after the full name, with the degree abbreviation coming after the comma.

> John Smith, MD, of Seattle, Washington.

See Appendix I: Professional Credentials and Academic Degrees

degrees, angle

See angles

degrees, burn

See classification systems

degrees, temperature

See temperature, temperature scales

deka-

Inseparable prefix meaning *10 units of a measure.*

To convert to basic unit, move decimal point one place to the right.

> 68 dekameters = 680 meters

Do not confuse with *deci-,* meaning *one-tenth of a unit.*

D

department names
See business names

depth
Express with numerals.

 4 inches deep
 3 mm in depth

derogatory remarks
See language to avoid

diabetes mellitus
The following information on the classification of diabetes mellitus is taken from the *Report of the Expert Committee on the Diagnosis and Classification of Diabetes Mellitus*, first published in 1997 and further modified since then (available through the American Diabetes Association, www.diabetes.org).

The two major changes made by the Expert Committee that affect medical transcriptionists are as follows:

1. The move away from the terms *insulin-dependent diabetes* and *non-insulin-dependent diabetes*. The report stressed that patients with any form of diabetes may require insulin at some stage of their disease but that such use of insulin does not, of itself, classify the disease.

2. The use of arabic rather than roman numerals for diabetes types.

type 1 and type 2 diabetes
The Expert Committee adopted the use of arabic numerals for diabetes types in order to improve communication, stating that it is too easy to confuse the roman numeral *II* for the arabic number *11*.

D

classification of diabetes mellitus

Type 1 diabetes (formerly *type I, insulin-dependent,* or *juvenile-onset diabetes*) is caused by ß-cell destruction. The two forms of type 1 diabetes are immune-mediated and idiopathic.

Type 2 diabetes (formerly *type II, non-insulin-dependent,* or *adult-onset diabetes*) is used for individuals who have insulin resistance and usually relative (rather than absolute) insulin deficiency.

The third class of diabetes comprises eight types and encompasses more than 45 specific diseases (examples of diseases for each type are shown in parentheses).

- genetic defects of ß-cell function (mitochondrial DNA)
- genetic defects in insulin action (leprechaunism)
- diseases of the exocrine pancreas (hemochromatosis)
- endocrinopathies (hyperthyroidism)
- drug- or chemical-induced (diazoxide)
- infections (cytomegalovirus)
- uncommon forms of immune-mediated diabetes (stiff man syndrome)
- other genetic syndromes sometimes associated with diabetes (Turner syndrome)

The fourth class is gestational diabetes mellitus (GDM), defined as any degree of glucose intolerance with its onset or first recognition during pregnancy.

The terms *impaired glucose tolerance* and *impaired fasting glucose tolerance* have been retained.

Classifications of diabetes mellitus in pregnancy include

- class A (gestational diabetes): Transient. *See* gestational diabetes *above*.
- class B: Initial onset after age 20, less than 10 years' duration, controlled by diet. Patient may become insulin-dependent during pregnancy but not need insulin after delivery.
- class C: Onset between ages 10 and 19. Insulin-dependent patient will need increased insulin during pregnancy but will likely return to pre-pregnancy dosage after delivery.
- class D: Onset before age 10, with more than 20 years' duration. Patient has hypertension, diabetic retinopathy, and peripheral vascular disease.
- class E: Patient has calcification of pelvic vessels.
- class F: Patient has diabetic nephropathy.

Infants of diabetic mothers may be described as

- LGA infants: large for gestational age. Infants of class A, B, and C mothers are apt to be LGA.
- SGA infants: small for gestational age. Infants of class D, E, and F mothers are apt to be SGA.

insulin-dependent and non-insulin-dependent diabetes

The terms *insulin-dependent diabetes (IDDM)* and *non-insulin-dependent diabetes (NIDM)* have been dropped because they are classifications based on treatment rather than etiology. However, they should be transcribed if dictated. The hyphens as shown here are retained by the Expert Committee.

insulin terminology

Express insulin concentrations as follows:

U40	contains 40 units per mL
U80	contains 80 units per mL
U100	contains 100 units per mL
U500	contains 500 units per mL

Insulin injections may be administered intravenously, intramuscularly, or subcutaneously.

preferred term	*also known as*
insulin injection	regular insulin, crystalline zinc
insulin injection, human	regular insulin, human

Insulin suspensions are administered only subcutaneously.

preferred term	*also known as*
insulin suspension, isophane	NPH insulin
insulin suspension, isophane, human	NPH insulin, human
insulin suspension, protamine zinc	PZI
insulin zinc suspension	lente insulin
insulin zinc suspension, extended	ultralente insulin
insulin zinc suspension, prompt	semilente insulin

diagnosis

abbreviations in diagnoses

Do not use abbreviations for diagnostic terms in document sections designating impression, admission diagnosis, discharge diagnosis, preoperative diagnosis, and postoperative diagnosis. If you cannot determine the meaning of a dictated abbreviation or acronym, transcribe it as dictated, then flag it, requesting that the originator explain the abbreviation or acronym.

D: Operation: Left BKA.
T: OPERATION: Left below-knee amputation.

While diagnostic terms must not be abbreviated in statements of diagnoses, some descriptive terms relating to the diagnosis may be abbreviated. Use abbreviations for units of measure.

> Laceration, 5 mm, left abdomen.

See abbreviations, acronyms, brief forms

numbering diagnoses

In section headings, when *diagnosis* is dictated, it may be changed to the plural form *diagnoses* if more than one is listed.

When only one diagnosis is given, it is preferable not to number it, even if a number is dictated, because the number gives the appearance that there are additional diagnoses. However, if there are several diagnoses it is preferable to number them even if numbers are not dictated.

> DIAGNOSIS
> Appendicitis.
>
> *preferred to*
>
> DIAGNOSIS
> 1. Appendicitis.

> D: Diagnosis: Appendicitis, history of "cabbage."
>
> T: DIAGNOSES
>   1. Appendicitis.
>   2. History of coronary artery bypass graft (CABG).

psychiatric diagnoses

A multiaxial system is often used in diagnosing psychiatric patients. Axis I is for all psychiatric disorders *except* mood disorders and mental retardation; axis II is for all personality disorders and mental retardation; axis III is for general medical conditions; axis IV, psychosocial and environmental problems; and axis V is an assessment of function, usually using the global assessment of functioning (GAF) scale. The following example demonstrates a

D

typical psychiatric diagnosis along with the applicable diagnostic codes found in the *Diagnostic and Statistical Manual of Mental Disorders, 4th edition (DSM-IV)*, which are consistent with ICD-9-CM and ICD-10 codes. (*See a brief discussion on* code, coding *elsewhere in this book.*)

Axis I	296.2	Major depressive disorder, single episode, severe, without psychotic features.
	305.0	Alcohol abuse.
Axis II	301.6	Dependent personality disorder.
Axis III	None.	
Axis IV		Threat of job loss.
Axis V	GAF = 3	(current)

"same"

Do not transcribe "same" when dictated for the discharge diagnosis (meaning same as admission diagnosis) or for the postoperative diagnosis (meaning same as preoperative diagnosis). Repeat the diagnosis in full.

> D: Admission diagnosis: Cholelithiasis.
> Discharge diagnosis: Same.
> T: ADMISSION DIAGNOSIS: Cholelithiasis.
> DISCHARGE DIAGNOSIS: Cholelithiasis.

> D: Preoperative diagnosis: uterine fibroid.
> Postoperative diagnosis: same.
> T: PREOPERATIVE DIAGNOSIS: Uterine fibroid.
> POSTOPERATIVE DIAGNOSIS: Uterine fibroid.

Beware of similar incomplete statements within the names of operations, and transcribe them in full.

> D: Preoperative diagnosis: left testicular hernia.
> T: PREOPERATIVE DIAGNOSIS: Left testicular hernia.

D: Operation performed: repair of same.

T: OPERATION PERFORMED: Repair of left testicular hernia.

differential diagnosis

When a patient presents with a group of symptoms and the diagnosis is unclear, the clinician may refer in the medical report to the *differential diagnosis* in order to compare and contrast the clinical findings of each. Although it consists of two or more possible diagnoses, the term *differential diagnosis* itself is singular and always takes a singular verb.

The differential diagnosis was...

diagonal (/)

See virgule

dictated but not read

Some originators or transcription supervisors direct that the statement "dictated but not read" (or a similar phrase such as "transcribed but not read" or "signed but not read") be entered at the end of a report in an attempt to waive the originator's responsibility to review the report and confirm its accuracy.

It is not appropriate for an MT to enter this statement because the MT can verify only that the report was transcribed; only the originator can verify that it was not read (and the latter is a fact that may change later). In addition, not reading records is a practice MTs should not encourage.

AAMT advises against the use of such phrases. A patient's report is authenticated when it is signed; the signature indicates that the report is accurate in the eyes of the authenticator, usually the report's originator. Medical transcriptionists must make every effort to be sure the report is transcribed accurately, but the final responsibility and authority lie with the originator.

D

If the MT is required to enter this statement, it is advisable to get the directive in writing, to document one's objections to it, and to retain that documentation should it be necessary to defend the action in the future.

dictation problems

A variety of dictation problems may occur, and medical transcriptionists' being alert to them is a form of risk management.

Watch for and correct obvious errors in dictation, including grammar, spelling, terminology, and style. When uncertain, draw suspected errors to the attention of the originator and/or supervisor.

When the change would be significant, particularly if it would influence medical meaning, leave a blank and flag it.

blank

Leave a blank when a dictated term, phrase, or abbreviation is unintelligible (whether due to equipment problems or mispronunciation) or cannot be confirmed through reasonable research; flag the report, briefly explaining why you left a blank, noting what the dictation sounds like, and asking for feedback for future reference.

Never "close up" the space where the unintelligible word, phrase, or sentence belongs, making it appear that a transcript is complete. Likewise, do not transcribe the questionable dictation, adding *[sic]* to indicate it is transcribed verbatim.

When the transcriptionist cannot determine how to edit the incorrect dictation properly, sometimes the best choice is to leave a blank and flag it. Appropriate use of blanks should prompt careful followup and contribute to patient care and risk management.

flag

A flag is a notation by the medical transcriptionist to the originator of a report, drawing attention to missing data, unclear dictation, errors in dictation, inconsistent dictation, equipment problems, potentially inflammatory remarks, etc. Flags contribute to risk management.

When flagging a printed report, cite the page, section, and line number. If the word or phrase is unfamiliar, note what it sounds like. If the term is inconsistent, briefly state why, e.g., "A left below-knee amputation is later referred to as right BK amputation. Which is correct?"

Similarly, flag medical inconsistencies you are unsure of, in order to permit review by the report's originator to assure accuracy.

Many systems now have methods in place to provide an "electronic flag," which should be noted as above, using the instructions for that particular system.

inconsistencies in dictation

A medical transcriptionist who identifies an inconsistency in dictation should resolve it if this can be done with competence and confidence. If the discrepancy cannot be resolved with certainty, the report should be flagged and brought to the attention of the supervisor or the report's originator for resolution.

> This 45-year-old male is status post hysterectomy. *(Either the patient is not male or he is status post another type of surgery.)*

See editing
  risk management

dictator

The person who, by voice, creates the document to be transcribed. The preferred term is *originator* or *author*.

See originator

die of, die from

Patients (and others) *die of*, not *from*, diseases, disorders, conditions, etc. Edit appropriately.

differ, different

To differ from means *to be unlike*. *To differ with* means *to disagree*. People and things are *different from*, not *different than*, one another.

differential blood cell count

See blood counts

dilation, dilatation

These two terms have become synonymous in meaning, each referring either to the act of expanding or the condition of being expanded, so transcribe as dictated.

Likewise, transcribe their verb forms, *dilate* and *dilatate*, as dictated.

> dilation and curettage
> *or* dilatation and curettage

dis-, dys-

Consult an appropriate reference (usually a medical dictionary) for guidance in determining which prefix is used with which term. Where either form is acceptable, use the preferred.

> disconjugate *preferred to* dysconjugate
> disequilibrium
> displacement
> disproportion

dysarthria

dyscrasia

dyskinesia

discharge summary

The report that recapitulates the reason for hospitalization, the significant findings, the procedures performed and treatment rendered, the condition of the patient on discharge, and the discharge plan is commonly known as the "discharge summary" or "clinical summary."

Typical content headings in a discharge summary include

chief complaint

admitting diagnosis

history of present illness

pertinent past history (past medical history)

physical examination on discharge

laboratory findings

hospital course

condition on discharge

discharge diagnoses (or final diagnoses)

disposition

prognosis

discharge instructions and medications

followup plans

See formats

Appendix A: Sample Reports

D

disease names

Lowercase disease names except for eponyms forming part of the name.

> sickle cell disease
> diabetes mellitus
> pelvic inflammatory disease
> Graves disease
> Lyme disease
> Parkinson disease
> parkinsonism

See eponyms

disk

Dictionaries and other reference works have long shown a lack of agreement about the spelling of this word. Some authorities prefer the spelling *disc* for references to the eye and *disk* for the spine. Others have an opposite preference.

We recommend the spelling *disk* for all anatomic and surgical references for this round, flat, regular, and regularly condensed plate of material.

There is classical support for this spelling. *Disk* is derived from the Greek *diskos* and came into our lexicon by way of medieval Latin *(discos)*, whose alphabet does not include a *k*. Other English words ending in *sk* with similar derivation include *ask, desk, kiosk, task*, and *whisk*. By comparison, there are very few English words that end in *sc*.

> optic disk
> L4-5 disk space
> diskectomy
> diskitis

distance

Express with numerals.

> She experiences shortness of breath after walking 4 blocks.

ditto marks (")

Do not use ditto marks to indicate *the same*; instead, repeat the term or phrase.

Do not use ditto marks as a symbol for *inches*, except in tables as a space-saving device.

> The infant was 22 inches long.
> *not* The infant was 22" long.

division symbol (÷)

Do not use this symbol except in tables and mathematical expressions.

dL

Abbreviation for *deciliter*.

Use with numerals.

Do not use periods.

Do not add *s* for plural.

Space between the numeral and the unit of measure.

> 20 dL

DNA

Abbreviation for *deoxyribonucleic acid*.

See genetics

D

DNR (do not resuscitate)

A DNR order is placed in a patient's chart when either the patient or the family has indicated that no emergency resuscitative measures are to be employed.

His status was changed to DNR yesterday.

Various labels are used for this type of directive, including *a comfort care order, a CPR order,* and *no-code.*

Because of his no-code status, the patient was not resuscitated and was pronounced dead at 0115 hours.

doctor, physician

The term *doctor* is a courtesy title that may be used by a medical or osteopathic doctor or by someone holding another type of doctoral degree, such as DC, DDS, PhD, JD, EdD, ND. Abbreviation: *Dr.* or *Dr* (the period is optional).

The term *physician* refers only to a medical or osteopathic doctor.

dollars and cents

Express exact amounts of dollars and cents with numerals, using a decimal point to separate dollars from cents.

$4.56

When written out, lowercase all terms.

a million dollars

amounts less than $1

Use numerals; spell out and lowercase *cents.*

Do not use the decimal form. Do not use the dollar sign ($). Do not use the cent sign (¢) except in tabular matter.

> 8 cents *not* $.08 *not* 8¢
>
> 20 cents *not* 20¢ *not* $.20
>
> *in tables:* 20¢ *not* .20¢ *not* $.20

However, in tables that include amounts over $1, those amounts that are less than $1 should include a zero preceding the decimal so that entries are consistent.

> $4.20
>
> $0.80

amounts over $1

Use the dollar sign ($) preceding the dollar amount, and separate dollars and cents by a decimal point.

Do not use a decimal following the dollar amount if cents are not included.

> $1.08
>
> $1.20
>
> $40 *(Note: not $40.00, unless listed in a column with other amounts that include cents.)*

subject-verb agreement

Monetary expressions take a singular verb when they are thought of as a sum, a plural verb when they are thought of as individual bills and coins.

> A million dollars is a lot of money.
>
> The 50 quarters were stacked on the dresser.

ranges
Repeat the dollar sign or cent sign but do not repeat the word forms.

Use *to* instead of a hyphen with dollar-sign or cent-sign forms.

> $4 to $5 *not* $4-$5
> 10¢ to 15¢ *not* 10¢-15¢

Use *to* with word forms.

> 4 to 5 dollars *not* 4-5 dollars
> 10 to 15 cents *not* 10-15 cents

possessive adjectives
Use *'s* or *s'*, whichever is appropriate, with units of money used as possessive adjectives.

> 1 dollar's worth
> 2 cents' worth

Do not use the possessive form with compound adjectives.

> a 2-dollar bill

international currencies
Sometimes it is important to distinguish US dollars from other currencies, such as Canadian dollars.

Note: There is no space between the letters and the *$* symbol.

> US$4.56
> Can$4.56

euro

The euro is the newly established (2002) currency for the European Union. Only time and usage will tell what the accepted plural forms will be. However, the official dossier from the European Union calls for the English plural of euro to be the same as the singular forms: *euro* and *cent*.

> 200 euro equal 200 cent

The official abbreviation for the *euro* is *EUR*.

dosage, dose

See drug terminology

double entendres

See language to avoid

Dr., Dr

Courtesy title for doctors. Use only for earned doctorates (medical or other), not honorary doctorates. The use of an ending period is optional.

> Dr. Brown
> Dr. C. Everett Koop
> *not* Dr. George W. Bush

Use *Dr.* not *Doctor* in salutations unless the salutation is directed to more than one doctor. Do not use *Drs.* as plural form in salutations; write out *Doctors* instead.

> Dear Dr. Watson:
> Dear Doctors Watson and Crick:

Do not use *Dr.* or *Doctor* when credentials are given.

> John Brown, MD
> *not* Dr. John Brown, MD

D

drug terminology
abbreviations and punctuation

Use lowercase abbreviations with periods for Latin abbreviations that are related to doses and dosages. Do not use abbreviations found on the "Dangerous Abbreviations" list from the Institute for Safe Medication Practices (**See** abbreviations, acronyms, brief forms *and* Appendix B: Dangerous Abbreviations).

Avoid using all capitals because they emphasize the abbreviation rather than the drug name. Avoid lowercase abbreviations without periods because some may be misread as words.

Do not translate.

abbreviation	Latin phrase	English translation
a.c.	ante cibum	before food
b.i.d.	bis in die	twice a day
gtt.	guttae	drops (better to spell out *drops*)
n.p.o.	nil per os	nothing by mouth
n.r.	non repetatur	do not repeat
p.c.	post cibum	after food
p.o.	per os	by mouth
p.r.n.	pro re nata	as needed
q.4 h.	quaque 4 hora	every 4 hours
q.h.	quaque hora	every hour
q.i.d.	quater in die	4 times a day
t.i.d.	ter in die	3 times a day
u.d.	ut dictum	as directed

Note: We have inserted a space after the numeral *4* in *q.4 h.* on the advice of the ISMP so that the number is more easily and clearly read.

Invalid Latin abbreviations such as *q.a.m. (every morning)* and mixed Latin and English abbreviations such as *q.4 hours (every 4 hours)* have become commonplace. However, as with all abbreviations, avoid those that are obscure (like *a.c.b.* for *before breakfast*) or dangerous. For example, *b.i.w.* is both obscure **and** dangerous. It is intended to mean *twice weekly* but it could be mistaken for *twice daily,* resulting in a dosage frequency seven times that intended.

Note: AAMT continues to discourage dropping periods in lowercase abbreviations that might be misread as words (for example, *bid* and *tid*). If you must drop the periods, use all capitals, but keep in mind that the overuse of capitals, particularly in relation to drug doses and dosages, would draw more attention to the capitalized abbreviations than to the drug names themselves.

Do not use commas to separate drug names from doses and instructions. In a series of drugs for each of which the dose and/or instructions are given, use commas to separate each complete entry. Exception: Use semicolons or periods when entries in the series have internal commas. Medications may also be listed vertically.

> The patient was discharged on Coumadin 10 mg daily.
>
> The patient was discharged on Carafate 1 g four times daily, 40 minutes after meals and at bedtime; bethanechol 25 mg p.o. q.i.d.; and Reglan 5 mg at bedtime on a trial basis.
>
> He was sent home on Biaxin 500 mg b.i.d., Atrovent inhaler 2 puffs q.i.d., and Altace 5 mg daily.

> CURRENT MEDICATIONS
> 1. Lescol 2 mg at bedtime.
> 2. DiaBeta 5 mg 1 q.a.m.
> 3. Aspirin 325 mg 1 daily.
> 4. Xanax 0.25 mg t.i.d. p.r.n.

dose and dosage

Dose means *the amount to be administered at one time,* or *total amount administered.*

D

Dosage means *regimen* and is usually expressed as a quantity per unit of time.

> dose: 5 mg
> dosage: 5 mg q.i.d.

Oral dosage forms include pills, tablets, and capsules. Liquid dosage forms may be solutions, emulsions, and suspensions. Topical dosage forms include suspensions or emulsions, such as ointments, creams, lotions, and gels. Other dosage forms include granules, powders, transdermal patches, ocular inserts, suppositories, subdermal pellets, solutions, sprays, drops, and injections.

The most common dosage route is oral for absorption through stomach or intestinal walls. Another common route is parenteral, such as intravenous, intramuscular, subcutaneous, intra-arterial, intradermal, intrathecal, and epidural. Other routes include topical, inhalation, rectal, vaginal, urethral, intramedullary, ocular, nasal, sublingual, and otic.

systems of measurement for drugs

Most pharmaceutical measurements for weight and volume are in the metric system. Although some units from the apothecary and avoirdupois systems remain in use, it should be noted that all elements of the apothecary system have been dropped from the compendium of the United States Pharmacopeia system (USP).

apothecary system

weight	liquid measure
1 grain (gr)	1 minim
1 scruple (20 gr)	1 fluidram (60 minims)
1 dram (60 gr)	1 fluidounce (8 fluidrams)
1 ounce (480 gr)	1 pint (16 fluidounces)
1 pound (5760 gr)	1 gallon (4 quarts or 8 pints)

Note: Either *fluidounce* or *fluid ounce* is an acceptable spelling.

avoirdupois system
1 grain
1 ounce (437.5 grains)
1 pound (16 ounces or 7000 grains)

brand name, trade name, trademark

The brand name is the manufacturer's name for a drug; it is the same as the trade name, trademark, or proprietary name. It may suggest a use or indication, and it often incorporates the manufacturer's name.

Capitalize brand names, trade names, and trademark names.

> Tagamet
> Bayer

Use of idiosyncratic capitalization is optional.

> pHisoHex *or* Phisohex

The trade name is a broader term than trademark, identifying the manufacturer but not the product.

Capitalize trade names.

> Dr. Scholl's

code name

The code name is the temporary designation for an as-yet-unnamed drug; it is assigned by the manufacturer. It may include a code number or code designation (number-letter combination).

chemical name

The chemical name describes the chemical structure of a drug. The

American Chemical Society, which is the internationally recognized source for such names, follows a set of guidelines established by chemists.

Do not capitalize chemical names.

> acetylsalicylic acid

generic name

The generic name is also known as the nonproprietary name, the established, official name for a drug. In the United States, it is created by the US Adopted Names Council (USAN). International nomenclature is coordinated by the World Health Organization.

Generic names are in the public domain; their use is unrestricted.

Do not capitalize generic names. When the generic name and brand name of a medication sound alike, use the generic spelling unless it is certain that the brand name is being referenced.

> aminophylline *(generic name)*
> *not* Aminophyllin *(brand name)*

isotope nomenclature

Used in reference to radioactive drugs.

When the element name, not the symbol, is used, place the isotope number on the line after the name in the same font and type size; do not superscript or subscript. Space between the element name and the isotope number. Do not hyphenate either the noun or the adjectival form.

> iodine 128
> technetium 99m

When the element symbol is used, place the isotope number as a superscript immediately before the symbol. Alternatively, use the following format: element symbol, space (**not** hyphen), isotope number (on the line), **or** avoid the nonsuperscript form by using the element name followed by the isotope number.

> ^{128}I *or* iodine 128
>
> ^{99m}Tc *or* Tc 99m *or* technetium 99m

For trademarked isotopes, follow the style of the manufacturer. In trademarks, the isotope is usually joined to the rest of the name by a hyphen; it may or may not be preceded by the element symbol.

> Glofil-125
>
> Hippuran I 131

interferons

A small class of glycoproteins that exert antiviral activity.

Use nonproprietary names as discussed below. For trade names and additional guidance, consult the USAN dictionary or other appropriate reference.

For general classes of compounds or single compounds, follow the lowercase interferon by the spelled-out Greek letter; use the Greek symbol in abbreviations. Note: *alfa* is the correct spelling in these terms, not *alpha*.

interferon alfa	IFN-α
interferon beta	IFN-ß
interferon gamma	IFN-γ

For individual, pure, identifiable compounds with nonproprietary names, add a hyphen, an arabic numeral, and a lowercase letter.

> interferon alfa-2a
> interferon alfa-2b
> interferon gamma-1a
> interferon gamma-1b

For names of mixtures of interferons from natural sources, add a hyphen, a lowercase *n*, and an arabic numeral.

> interferon alfa-n1
> interferon alfa-n2

multiple-drug regimens

Abbreviations for multiple-drug regimens are acceptable if widely used and readily recognized.

> MOPP (methotrexate, vincristine sulfate, prednisone, and procarbazine)

vitamins

Lowercase *vitamin*, capitalize the letter designation, and use arabic numerals (in subscript form if available). Do not use a hyphen or space between the letter and numeral.

> vitamin B12 *or* vitamin B_{12}
> B12 vitamin *or* B_{12} vitamin

vitamin	*drug name*
vitamin B1	thiamine hydrochloride
vitamin B2	riboflavin
vitamin B6	pyridoxine hydrochloride
vitamin B12	cyanocobalamin

vitamin C	ascorbic acid
vitamin D2	ergocalciferol
vitamin D3	cholecalciferol
vitamin K1	phytonadione
vitamin K3	menadione

See Appendix B: Dangerous Abbreviations

Dukes classification of carcinoma
See cancer classifications

each

Singular term, so it takes a singular verb.

> Each patient was complaining of...
>
> Each of the tests was repeated x3.

ECG, EKG

Acceptable abbreviations for *electrocardiogram*, *electrocardiography*, and *electrocardiographic*.

Transcribe either *ECG* or *EKG*, as dictated.

See cardiology

editing

Verbatim transcription of dictation is seldom possible. MTs should prepare reports that are as correct, clear, consistent, and complete as can be reasonably expected, without imposing their personal style on those reports. Tools for editing include dictionaries, word books, style books, textbooks, grammar software, other teaching materials, experts, and experience.

> D: The patient developed a puffy right eye that was felt to be secondary to an insect bite by the ophthalmologist.
>
> T: The patient developed a puffy right eye; this was felt by the ophthalmologist to be secondary to an insect bite.

> D: CAT scan showed there was nothing in the brain but sinusitis.
>
> T: CAT scan of the brain showed only sinusitis.

Editing is inappropriate in medical transcription when it alters information without the editor's being certain of the appropriateness or accuracy of the change, when it second-guesses the originator, when it deletes appropriate and/or essential information, and when it tampers with the originator's style.

Edit grammar, punctuation, spelling, and similar dictation errors as necessary to achieve clear communication. Likewise, edit slang words and phrases, incorrect terms, incomplete phrases, English or medical inconsistencies, and inaccurate phrasing of laboratory data.

> D: temp
> T: temperature
>
> D: Operation: Teflon tube.
> T: Operation: Teflon tube insertion.

When transcribing dictation by those who speak English as a second language, edit obvious errors, following the general guidelines for editing. It is not necessary or recommended that such dictation be rewritten; rather, the physician's basic style should be retained.

Transcription businesses and departments should establish clear policies and instructions on how to deal with inappropriate language or inflammatory remarks in dictation. Medical transcriptionists should check with their supervisors to determine the rules for editing or omitting such language and remarks from transcription.

Institutional policy and originator preference are major factors in decisions to edit. To the extent that editing is acceptable in your setting and to the originator, the following guidelines for editing are recommended.

For additional guidelines and examples, **See** *other topics in this book, in particular* dictation problems *and* language to avoid.

clarifying content

Refer to the patient's record to clarify or correct content in dictation. If the record is not available, draw attention to errors or potentially confusing entries for which you do not have sufficient information to make corrections.

leaving blanks

Leave a blank space in a report rather than guessing what was meant or transcribing unclear or obviously incorrect dictation. Flag the report to draw attention to the blank.

flagging reports

When flagging a report to draw attention to unclear or incorrect dictation, cite the page, section, and line number, tagging the error on paper or electronically. If the word or phrase is unfamiliar, note what it sounds like. If the term is inconsistent, briefly state why, e.g., "A left below-knee amputation is later referred to as right BK amputation. Which is correct?"

Similarly, draw attention to medical inconsistencies you have corrected, in order to encourage the originator's review to assure accuracy.

negative findings

Never delete negative or normal findings if dictated. To do so is altering the dictation as well as the medical record. *See* negative findings.

speech recognition and editing

The computerized translation by a speech recognition engine of dictated material results in text that usually needs considerable editing. This is sometimes done by the originator but more often by a person with the medical knowledge and language skills of a medical transcriptionist, who ideally will review the text while listening to the originator's voice file, checking for errors and inconsistencies. The same editing guidelines that apply to medical transcription apply to editing the text resulting from speech-recognized dictation.

See dictation problems
　　language to avoid
　　negative findings

EEG

Abbreviation for *electroencephalography*, *electroencephalograph*, and *electroencephalogram*.

See electroencephalographic terms

effect

See affect, effect

either

Meaning one or the other.

Replace *both* with *either* if the meaning is one or the other, **not** both. Replace *either* with *both* if that is the meaning intended.

> D: There were wounds on either leg.
> T: There were wounds on both legs.

either...or, neither...nor

See conjunctions

EKG, ECG

Acceptable abbreviations for *electrocardiogram*, *electrocardiography*, and *electrocardiographic*.

Transcribe either *EKG* or *ECG*, as dictated.

See cardiology

electroencephalographic terms

EEG

Abbreviation for *electroencephalogram, electroencephalography,* and *electroencephalograph.*

symbols for electrodes

Use capital letters to refer to anatomic areas.

Use subscript lowercase letters to refer to relative electrode positions. Use subscript odd numbers to refer to electrodes placed on the left. Subscript even numbers refer to those on the right; subscript *z* refers to midline (zero) electrodes. If subscripts are not available, place the lowercase letters, numbers, and *z* on the line, adjacent to the capital letter and to each other, or spell out the terms.

A1, A2	A_1, A_2	earlobe electrodes
Cz, C3, C4	C_z, C_3, C_4	central electrodes
F7, F8	F_7, F_8	anterior temporal electrodes
Fpz, Fp1, Fp2	F_{pz}, F_{p1}, F_{p2}	frontal pole; prefrontal electrodes
Fz, F3, F4	F_z, F_3, F_4	frontal electrodes
Oz, O1, O2	O_z, O_1, O_2	occipital electrodes
Pg1, Pg2	P_{g1}, P_{g2}	nasopharyngeal electrodes
Pz, P3, P4	P_z, P_3, P_4	parietal electrodes
T3, T4	T_3, T_4	midtemporal electrodes
T5, T6	T_5, T_6	posterior temporal electrodes

frequency

Express in cycles per second (*c/s* or *cps*) or hertz *(Hz).*

16 c/s *or* 16 cps *or* 16 Hz

some terms commonly used in EEG reports

alert, drowsy, and sleeping states	photic stimulation
alpha range	rhythmic activity
alpha rhythm	sharp elements
alpha waves	sharp waves
amplitude	sleep spindles
artifact	slow transients
background rhythm	slow waves
beta rhythms	spike and dome complex
bisynchronous	spike and wave pattern
central sleep spindles	spikes
cycles per second (c/s, cps)	spindles
delta brush	Standard International lead placements
delta spikes	symmetrical activity
delta waves	synchronous
frontal sharp transient	theta activity
hyperventilation	theta frequency
lambda rhythm	21-channel recording
lateralizing focus	vertex waves
mu pattern	voltage
occipital driving	wave bursts
paroxysmal, paroxysms	

elliptical construction

A construction in which one or more words have been left out but are understood.

Use a semicolon to separate the elliptical construction from what precedes it. A comma is acceptable if the elliptical construction does not require other internal punctuation.

The white count was abnormal; the red, normal.
or The white count was abnormal, the red normal.

endocrinology

See diabetes mellitus

hormones

end-of-line word division

See word division

eponyms

Names of entities—e.g., diseases, anatomic structures, operations, or tests—derived from the names of persons or places.

Homans sign

Lyme disease

Down syndrome

capitalization

Capitalize eponyms but not the common nouns, adjectives, and prefixes that accompany them.

Do not capitalize words derived from eponyms.

ligament of Treitz

red Robinson catheter

non-Hodgkin lymphoma

Parkinson disease *but* parkinsonism

Cushing syndrome *but* cushingoid

plurals

Do not use an apostrophe in the plural forms of eponyms.

Babinskis were negative.

possessive form

AAMT first advocated dropping the possessive form of eponyms in 1990. We adopted this standard because it promotes consistency and clarity. More recently, *The AMA Manual of Style* (1998), *Stedman's Medical Dictionary* (2000), and *Dorland's Illustrated Medical Dictionary* (2000), have acknowledged the trend away from the possessive form.

It is important to note, however, that use of the possessive form remains an acceptable alternative if dictated and/or if indicated as the preference by employer or client.

> Apgar score
> Babinski sign
> Down syndrome
> Gram stain
> Hodgkin lymphoma

In awkward constructions, such as when the noun following the eponym is omitted, the possessive form becomes preferred.

> The patient's husband suffers from Alzheimer's.

equal

This term does not have comparative or superlative forms. Thus, *more equal* and *most equal* are incorrect forms. *Equitable* is probably the term intended in such constructions.

> A more equitable solution to the problem would be...
> *not* A more equal solution to the problem would be...

equal, equal to (=)

Do not use the symbol except in tables and mathematical presentations.

equally

Not *equally as.*

> The twins were equally developed.
> *not* The twins were equally as developed.

equator readings

Use a colon to express equator readings.

> Sclerotomy drainage was done at the 8:30 equator.

Sometimes, the term *equator* or a substitute term (e.g., *position*) may not be dictated. Add the term if its absence may confuse the reader (who may interpret it as clock time rather than position).

> D: Sclerotomy drainage was done at 8:30.
> T: Sclerotomy drainage was done at the 8:30 position.

equipment terms

Capitalize brand (proprietary) names of equipment, and lowercase adjectives and nouns that accompany them.

Do not use trademark symbols (™ or ®).

Lowercase generic (nonproprietary) names.

> American Optical photocoagulator

model numbers

Use arabic numerals to express model numbers of instruments, equipment, etc.

E

Lowercase *model.*

Use capital or lowercase letters, the number symbol *(#)*, hyphens, and spaces as they are used by the manufacturer. If not known, use capital letters and no hyphens or spaces, except as dictated.

> model C453
> model #8546

serial numbers

Use arabic numerals to express serial numbers of instruments, equipment, etc.

Lowercase *serial.*

Use capital or lowercase letters, the number symbol *(#)*, hyphens, and spaces as they are used by the manufacturer. If not known, use capital letters and no hyphens or spaces, except as dictated.

> serial #A185403

esophagram, esophagogram

The terms are used interchangeably.

Transcribe as dictated.

ex-

Use a hyphen to form *ex-* compounds when *ex-* means *former* and precedes a noun that can stand on its own. Otherwise, *ex-* is joined directly to the following term (without a hyphen), with the usual exceptions for prefixes applying.

ex-husband
ex-president
excretion
exfoliate

exam

Acceptable brief form of *examination* when dictated, except as a heading.

The physical exam was negative.

PHYSICAL EXAMINATION
HEENT
Head normal.
Neck supple.

Do not use the brief form if the expanded form is dictated.

D: physical examination
T: physical examination *not* physical exam

exclamation point (!)

Use an exclamation point to express great surprise, incredulity, or other forceful emotion or comment. Use it primarily in direct quotations; avoid it otherwise in medical transcription except in rare instances. Use a comma or period for mild exclamations.

The patient loudly insisted, "You have already examined me!"
"No," I replied quietly but firmly.

exclamation point (!)

Place the exclamation point inside the ending quotation mark if the material being quoted is an exclamatory statement. Never combine the exclamation point with a period, comma, question mark, or other exclamation point.

"Stop!" the patient cried as I approached her with the needle and syringe.
not "Stop!," the patient cried...

The patient insisted, "You have already examined me!"
not The patient insisted, "You have already examined me!".

Place the exclamation point before the closing parenthesis when an exclamatory statement is placed within parentheses.

The patient insisted I had already examined her (I had not!) and refused to cooperate.

Place the exclamation point outside the closing parenthesis when the entire sentence (not just the parenthetical matter) is an exclamation.

What a fiasco (the patient left before I finished my exam)!

expendable words

Redundant words or phrases that not only can be omitted without changing the meaning, but whose omission improves readability.

Avoid overuse and misuse, but the following are acceptable if transcribed as dictated.

it goes without saying
needless to say
in other words
it was shown that
quite
very
rather

For the following phrases, drop the redundant words (those in italics).

12 noon

12 midnight

a.m. *o'clock*

a.m. *in the morning*

at this *point in* time

basic *fundamental*

blood pressure *reading*

consensus *of opinion*

e.g., *for example*

etc., *and so forth*

i.e., *that is*

my *personal* view

p.m. *in the evening*

round *in shape*

small *in size*

sum *total*

two halves

yellow *in color*

exponents

Exponents are generally superscripted, but if superscripting is not available, use appropriate abbreviations (*cu* or *sq*) instead. Avoid placing the numerals on the line, since the terms are not easily read in this form.

10^5 *or* 10 to the 5th

4 cm^2 *or* 4 sq cm (*rather than* cm2)

8 mm^3 *or* 8 cu mm (*rather than* mm3)

F

FAB classification

See cancer classifications

family relationship names

Capitalize words that denote family relationships only when they are within quotations and they precede the person's name or when they stand alone as a substitute for the name.

> Family history: She reported, "My Grandmother Ross raised me."

> He said, "Every morning Mother told me..."
> He said, "Every morning my mother told me..."
> He said every morning his mother told him...

When the originator refers to a patient's relative by a familiar term, edit to the formal term. (Note: Some physicians, in particular pediatricians, prefer the use of the informal term, e.g., *mom*, when referring to a patient's parents.)

> D: The child stayed in bed all day, but mom says there was no fever.
> T: ...but his mother says there was no fever.

farther, further

Farther refers to physical distance; *further*, to extension of time or degree.

> He drove farther than planned.
> He needs further care before discharge.

 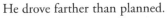

F

fax

Widely accepted and preferred brief form for *facsimile*.

Do not capitalize; do not use periods. Plural: *faxes*.

Also used as a verb: *fax, faxes, faxed, faxing*.

> His previous physician faxed the report to me.

fellow, Fellow

Lowercase when referring to academic or specialty position.

> He is a fellow of the American Academy of Orthopaedic Surgeons.

A physician's credentials may include a fellowship. In the following example, the doctor is a fellow of the American College of Physicians-American Society of Internal Medicine (ACP-ASIM).

> Jefferey Smith, MD, FACP

Capitalize when used in a formal signature or address.

> Jean P. Smith, MD
> Clinical Fellow, Oncology

Lowercase for casual usage.

> All 3 fellows agreed with my diagnosis.

See Appendix I: Professional Credentials and Academic Degrees

fever

See temperature, temperature scales

fewer, less

Fewer refers to a number of individuals or things. *Less* refers to a single amount or mass. Do not use the terms interchangeably.

> He has fewer complaints than previously.
>
> He has less pain than previously.

Use *less* for quantities accompanied by a unit of measure because the quantity plus unit is considered a collective noun.

> The lesion was less than 5 mm in diameter.

fingerbreadth

Plural form is *fingerbreadths* not *fingersbreadth*.

flag

See dictation problems

fluctuance, fluctuation

Fluctuation and *fluctuance* are synonymous. Note: "Fluctuants" is not a word.

The adjectival form is *fluctuant*.

Fluctuance was not found in dictionaries until 2000 when it was added to the 27th edition of *Stedman's Medical Dictionary* as a secondary spelling for *fluctuation*.

fluidounce, fluid ounce

Either form is acceptable.

followthrough, follow through

For the noun and adjective forms, AAMT prefers *followthrough*; the hyphenated form *follow-through* is an acceptable alternative.

> Because of poor followthrough by the caretaker, the patient became noncompliant. *(noun)*

The two-word form *follow through* is the only correct choice for the verb form.

> He promises to follow through with his doctor's suggestions. *(verb)*

followup, follow up

Use *followup* for the noun and adjective forms (the hyphenated form, *follow-up* is an acceptable alternative).

> The patient did not return for followup. *(noun)*

> In followup visits, she appeared to improve. *(adjective)*

For the verb, the two-word form *follow up* is the only correct choice.

> We will follow up with regular return visits. *(verb)*

font

A particular size and style for a printed character. The style and size of the font influences line length, which in turn can affect productivity measurement in transcription.

See Appendix E: Full Disclosure in Medical Transcription

HINT: To test whether the correct form is one word or two, try changing the tense or number. If one or more letters must be added, the correct form is two words.

We will follow up.

tense change >>

We followed up.

(*Followedup* is not a word, so *followed up* must be two words.)

We follow up.

number change >>

He follows up.

(*Followsup* is not a word, so *follows up* must be two words.)

F

food

Lowercase most food names.

>   baked beans

Capitalize brand names and trademarks but not the nouns or adjectives that accompany them.

>   Campbell's baked beans

Capitalize most proper nouns or adjectives used in food names, except when the meaning does not require the proper noun or adjective. The same rule applies to foreign names. Check appropriate references (dictionaries or the US Trademark website: www.uspto.gov/web/menu/tm.html) for guidance.

>   Boston baked beans
>   french fries
>   graham crackers
>   Manhattan cocktail
>   melba toast

foot

Basic unit of length in the measuring system used in the United States. Equal to 12 inches. The metric equivalent is 30.48 cm.

To convert to approximate centimeters, multiply by 30; for exact conversion, multiply by 30.48.

>   5 feet = 150 cm *(approximate)*

To convert to approximate meters, multiply by 0.3; for exact conversion, multiply by 0.3048.

>   5 feet = 1.5 m *(approximate)*

F

Write out; do not use abbreviation *(ft.)* or symbol *(')* except in tables.

Express accompanying quantities as numerals.

Do not use a comma or other punctuation with units of the same dimension.

> 10 feet 11 inches
> 5 pounds 4 ounces

for example

Latin equivalent is *exempli gratia*, abbreviated *e.g.*

Place a comma before and after both the English and Latin forms.

> Medical transcription requires knowledge in many areas, e.g., medical terminology, technology, and medicolegal issues.

See Latin abbreviations

foreign terms

Do not italicize foreign abbreviations, words, and phrases used in medical reports.

Capitalize, punctuate, and space according to the standards of the language of origin.

Omit accent marks except in proper names or where current usage retains them.

> cul-de-sac
> en masse
> facade
> i.e.
> in vivo

naive

peau d'orange

resume

Do not translate foreign words or abbreviations unless the originator translates them.

F

formats

While various institutional formats are acceptable, standardized formats for many report types have been developed by the Healthcare Informatics committee of ASTM in a standard called *E2184, Standard Specification for Healthcare Document Formats*, which specifies the requirements for the sections and subsections, and their arrangement, in an individual's healthcare documents. Some of the formatting suggestions in this book—in particular H&Ps and similar reports—are consistent with those published in the ASTM standard.

Block format is preferred (all lines flush left) for all reports, as well as for correspondence, but institutional and client preferences may vary and should prevail.

margins

Leave half-inch to one-inch margins, top and bottom, left and right.

Ragged-right margins are preferred over right-justified margins, with all lines flush left (block format).

To enhance readability, avoid end-of-line hyphenation except for terms with pre-existing hyphens.

paragraphs

Use paragraphs to separate narrative blocks within sections. In general, start new paragraphs as dictated except when such paragraphing is excessive (some originators start a new paragraph with every sentence or two) or inadequate (some originators dictate an entire lengthy report in one paragraph).

F

section and subsection headings

Title reports and report sections as dictated, unless you are following a standardized format. Institutional and client preferences should prevail.

Use all capitals for major section headings. Use initial capitals for subsection headings.

Avoid underlining because it diminishes readability.

List chief complaint, diagnoses, preoperative diagnoses, postoperative diagnoses, names of operations, and similar entries vertically. If the originator numbers some but not all items, be consistent and number all or none. When a single diagnosis is referred to as "number one," it is better to delete the number so that the reader is not led to believe that additional entries are missing.

Obvious headings that are not dictated may be inserted, but this is not required. If the originator moves in and out of sections, insert the information into the appropriate sections. (Headings may be omitted where appropriate.)

Double-space between major sections of reports.

List subsection headings vertically to assist the reader in identifying particular subsections.

Do not use abbreviations or brief forms in headings except for such widely used and readily recognizable abbreviations as *HEENT*, if dictated.

Place the content on the next line following the section or subsection heading, if possible. The ASTM "Formats" standard calls for an extra line space between subheadings, as in the following example.

HEENT
Within normal limits.

Thorax and Lungs
No rales or rhonchi.

Cardiovascular
No murmurs.

When the information following the section or subsection heading continues on the same line, use a colon (not a hyphen or a dash) after each heading.

HEENT: Within normal limits.
THORAX AND LUNGS: No rales or rhonchi.
CARDIOVASCULAR: No murmurs.

Capitalize the word following the heading, whether or not a colon follows the heading. Exception: When quantity and unit of measure immediately follow a heading such as *estimated blood loss*, use numerals.

LUNGS: Within normal limits.
ESTIMATED BLOOD LOSS: 10 mL.

End each entry with a period unless it is a date or the name of a person.

ANESTHESIOLOGIST: Sharon Smith, MD
ANESTHESIA: General.

signature block

Enter the signature block four lines below the final line of text, flush left. Use the originator's full name. If a title is given, place it directly below the originator's name; use initial capitals, unless institutional style calls for all caps. Note: Signature lines are often preformatted; in that case, leave as formatted.

Ruth T. Gross, MD
Chief of Pediatrics

F

initials of originator and transcriptionist at end of transcript

It is common practice to include originator and transcriptionist initials at the end of each report. When used, enter the initials flush left two lines below last line of text. Use either all capitals or all lowercase letters for both sets of initials, with a colon or virgule between them. Do not use periods.

Do not include academic degrees, professional credentials, or titles.

> RH:ST *or* rh:st
> RH/ST *or* rh/st

Some facilities may choose to identify the originators and MTs by other identifiers, such as a number or a number-letter combination, and system-generated reports may enter these identifiers automatically along with date, time, and place stamps.

> Dictated: D283, 02/02/02, 2:35 p.m., Indianapolis, IN
> Transcribed: T149, 02/02/02, 11:40 p.m., LaFayette, IN

time and date stamp

For the sake of an audit trail, it is common practice to include the date and time of dictation and transcription at the end of each report. Enter the date and time flush left below the initials of the originator and transcriptionist. Use colons for the time unless military time is the preferred format.

Note: Identification of the place of dictation and transcription may be required as well.

> D: 02/02/02, 11:40 p.m., LaFayette, IN
> T: 2/3/02, 8:45 a.m., Springfield, MO

continuation pages

When a transcript is longer than one page, enter *continued* at the bottom of each printed page prior to the last, and repeat the patient's name and medical record number, the page number, the type and date of report on each continuation page. Additional identifying data may be noted, according to the employer's or client's preference.

Do not carry a single line of a report onto a continuation page. Do not allow a continuation page to include only the signature block and the data following it.

When the printing is done by someone other than the medical transcriptionist, or when it is programmed into the system, these guidelines should still be followed.

See audit trails
correspondence
word division
Appendix A: Sample Reports

formula

A mathematical or chemical formula may include a combination of numbers and symbols. Plural: *formulas*.

See chemical nomenclature

Fort

Abbreviate or spell out *Fort* in proper names according to common or preferred usage related to the entity in question. Of course, spell out and lowercase generic uses.

Fort Collins
Ft. Laramie
The children were playing in a makeshift fort when the accident occurred.

F

fractions

Use numerals for fractional measurements preceding a noun. Join the fraction to the unit of measure with a hyphen, whether you use the symbol for the fraction or create it with whole numbers.

A ¼-inch incision was made.
A 3/4-pound tumor was removed.
The abdomen shows a 4-1/4-inch scar.

Spell out fractional measurements that are less than one when they do not precede a noun.

The tumor weighed three quarters of a pound.

Place a hyphen between numerator and denominator when neither contains a hyphen.

one-fourth empty
two-thirds full
but
one forty-eighth *or* 1/48
twenty-three thirty-eighths *or* 23/38

Hyphenate fractions when they are written out and used as adjectives; do not hyphenate those written out and used as nouns.

one-half normal saline
one third of the calf

The patient cut the medication in half because she did not tolerate it well.

F

ages

Use numerals for fractions in ages.

> 3 years old
>
> 3-1/2-year-old child

dimensions

Use numerals for fractions in pairs of dimensions.

> The wound was 4-1/2 x 3-1/2 inches.

tables

Use numerals to express fractions in tables.

mixed fractions

If you cannot create reduced-size fractions that can be placed directly following whole numbers, then use the "numeral-virgule-numeral" style, placing a hyphen between the whole number and the fraction.

> 1½ weeks *or* 1-1/2 weeks
>
> 5½-year-old girl *or* 5-1/2-year-old girl

fracture-dislocation

Use a hyphen, as indicated.

> *See* compound words
> orthopedics

fraternal organizations and service clubs

Capitalize proper names and those designating membership.

> Rotary Club
> Rotarian

French, french

Capitalize when referring to the country, its people, or its culture.

French-speaking

Do not capitalize such usage as *french fries, french door, french cuff.*

French Canadian

Do not hyphenate.

See sociocultural designations

French scale

Sizing system for catheters, sounds, and other tubular instruments. Each unit is approximately 0.33 mm in diameter.

Precede by *#* or *No.* if the word "number" is dictated.

Capitalize *French.*

5-French catheter

#5-French catheter

catheter, size 5 French

Keep in mind that *French* is linked to diameter size and is not the eponymic name of an instrument. Thus, it is a 15-French catheter, not a French catheter, size 15.

g

Abbreviation for *gram*. Preferred to *gm*, which is still acceptable. Neither form uses a final period.

> 4 g *preferred to* 4 gm

See gram

gallon

Equal to 4 quarts or 128 fluidounces. Metric equivalent is approximately 3.8 liters.

To convert to liters, multiply by 3.8.

Do not abbreviate *(gal)* except in tables.

> 4 gallons = 15.2 liters

gay

Term commonly used for a homosexual person, whether male or female, although many gay females prefer the term *lesbian*. Do not capitalize. Noun and adjective forms are the same.

genetics

chromosomal terms

There are 46 chromosomes in human cells, occurring in pairs and numbered 1 through 22, plus the sex chromosomes, an X and a Y in males and two X's in females. The non-sex chromosomes are also called autosomes.

group designations

Refer to chromosomes by number or by group.

chromosome	group
1-3	A
4, 5	B
6-12, X	C
13-15	D
16-18	E
19, 20	F
21, 22, Y	G

chromosome 16

a chromosome in group E

a group-E chromosome

trisomy: an extra chromosome in any one of the autosomes or either sex chromosome

trisomy D: an extra chromosome in a group-D chromosome, either the 13th, 14th, or 15th chromosome

trisomy 21: an extra 21st chromosome (Down syndrome)

A plus or minus in front of the chromosome number means there is either an extra chromosome or an absent chromosome within that pair.

trisomy 21 = female karyotype: 47,XX +21

The plus or minus following the chromosome number means that part of the chromosome is either extra or missing.

cri du chat syndrome = male karyotype: 46,X6 5p-

arms

Each chromosome has a short arm and a long arm. The short arm is designated by a *p*, the long arm by a *q*, immediately following the chromosome number (no space between). Each arm is divided into regions (from 1 to 4); place the region number immediately following the arm designation. Regions are divided into bands, again joined without a space. If a subdivision is identified, it follows a decimal point placed immediately after the band number.

20p	20th chromosome, short arm
20p1	20th chromosome, short arm, region 1
20p11	20th chromosome, short arm, region 1, band 1
20p11.23	20th chromosome, short arm, region 1, band 1, subdivision 23

A translocation occurs when a segment normally found in a certain arm of a chromosome appears in a different location; it may be written as a small *t* with the *from* and *to* sites in parentheses, e.g., t(14q21q), meaning from long arm of 14 to long arm of 21. A more complex designation such as t(2;6)(q34;p12) means from region 3 band 4 of the long arm of chromosome 2 to region 1 band 2 of the short arm of chromosome 6. The chromosome numbers appear in a separate set of parentheses from the arm, region, and band information.

A ring chromosome is one that has pieces missing from the end of each arm, and the two arms have joined at the ends.

G

bands

Use capital letters to refer to chromosome bands, which are elicited by special staining methods.

band	*stain*
C bands *or* C-banding	constitutive heterochromatin
G bands *or* G-banding	Giemsa
N bands *or* N-banding	nucleolar organizing region
Q bands *or* Q-banding	quinacrine
R bands *or* R-banding	reverse-Giemsa

karyotype

Describes an individual's chromosome complement: the number of chromosomes plus the sex chromosomes present in that individual. Place a comma (without spacing) between the chromosome number and the sex chromosome. Use a virgule to indicate more than one karyotype in an individual.

normal human karyotypes:	46,XX (female)
	46,XY (male)

some abnormal karyotypes:	47,XXY
	45,X0
	48,XXX
	45,X/46,XX

genes

Molecular units of heredity; their locations are called loci. A gene's main form and its locus have the same symbol, usually an abbreviation for the gene name or a quality of the gene. The symbol usually consists of 3 or 4 characters, all capitals, or all capitals and an arabic numeral, all on the line (no superscripts or subscripts). Do not use hyphens or spaces. Italics are used in formal publications, but regular type is preferred in medical transcription.

CF	cystic fibrosis
G6PD	glucose-6-phosphate dehydrogenase
HPRT	hypoxanthine phosphoriboxyltransferase
PHP	panhypopituitarism

Alleles are alternative forms of genes. To express their symbols, add an asterisk and the allele designation to the gene symbol. Italics are used in formal publications, but regular type is preferred in medical transcription.

HBB*6V

biochemical constituents

The biochemical constituents of genetics include deoxyribonucleic acid, ribonucleic acid, and the amino acids.

deoxyribonucleic acid (DNA)

DNA includes the bases thymine (T), cytosine (C), adenine (A), and guanine (G). DNA contains the genetic code and is found in the chromosomes of humans and animals. DNA expressions and their abbreviations include

complementary DNA	cDNA
double-stranded DNA	dsDNA
single-stranded DNA	ssDNA

ribonucleic acid (RNA)

RNA includes the bases cytosine, adenine, and guanine, and uracil (U). RNA is functionally associated with DNA. RNA expressions and their abbreviations include

heterogeneous RNA	hnRNA
messenger RNA	mRNA
ribosomal RNA	rRNA
small nuclear RNA	snRNA
transfer RNA	tRNA

G

amino acids of proteins
Write out in text. In tables, use three-letter or one-letter abbreviations.

phenylalanine	Phe	F
proline	Pro	P
tryptophan	rp	W

oncogenes
Viral genes in certain retroviruses.

Express as three-letter lowercase terms derived from names of associated viruses. Italics are used in formal publications, but regular type is used in medical transcription.

abl

mos

sis

src

The prefix *v-* *(virus)* or *c-* (*cellular* or *chromosomal counterpart*) indicates the location of the oncogene. The *c*-prefixed oncogenes are also known as proto-oncogenes and may be alternatively expressed in all capitals, without the prefix. Italics are used in formal publications, but regular type is preferred in medical transcription. Note: The prefix is never italicized.

genus and species names
A genus includes species whose broad features are alike in organization but different in detail.

A species is a group of individuals that can interbreed and produce fertile offspring. A species name is usually preceded by its genus name.

capitalization

Always capitalize genus names and their abbreviated forms when they are accompanied by a species name.

Always lowercase species names.

> Haemophilus influenzae
> Escherichia coli
> Staphylococcus aureus

Lowercase genus names used in plural and adjectival forms and when used in the vernacular, for example, when they stand alone (without a species name).

> staphylococcus
> group B streptococcus
> staphylococci
> staphylococcal infection
> staph infection
> strep throat

-osis, -iasis

The suffixes *-osis* and *-iasis* indicate disease caused by a particular class of infectious agents or types of infection.

Lowercase terms formed with these suffixes.

> amebiasis
> dermatophytosis

abbreviations

In a second reference to a genus-species term, the genus name may be abbreviated as a single letter without a period. (Note: Some references use a period, but AAMT recommends dropping it.) A longer abbreviation may be used to avoid confusion.

> S aureus
> *or* Staph aureus

Do not abbreviate the species name even if the genus name is abbreviated.

> D: H flu
> T: H influenzae

italics

In medical transcription, do not use italics for genus and species names.

geographic names
abbreviations

State and territory names may be abbreviated when they are preceded by a city name, and country names may be abbreviated when preceded by a city, state, or territory name.

> Orlando, FL
> Washington, DC

Do not abbreviate names of states, territories, countries or similar units within reports when they stand alone.

> The patient moved here 3 years ago from Canada.

However, abbreviations **may** be used in addresses, and **should** be used when addressing envelopes.

G

capitalization

Capitalize names of political divisions such as streets, cities, towns, counties, states, countries; topographic names, e.g., mountains, rivers, oceans, islands; and accepted designations for regions.

> the Bay Area
> Great Britain
> Lake Wobegon
> the Middle East
> Wallingford Avenue
> Yosemite National Park

Capitalize common nouns that are an official part of a proper name; lowercase them when they stand alone.

> Philippine Islands
> the islands

Capitalize compass directions when they are part of the geographic name. ***See*** north, south, east, west.

> East Timor

Capitalize geographic names used as eponyms.

> Lyme disease

Do not capitalize words derived from geographic names when they have a special meaning.

> india ink
> plaster of paris
> french fries

G

foreign places

Use primary spelling as indicated in a recognized English dictionary.

commas

In text, use a comma before and after the state name preceded by a city name, or a country name preceded by a state or city name.

> The patient is from San Francisco and moved to Modesto, California, 15 years ago.

> The patient returned from a business trip to Paris, France, the week prior to admission.

greater, Greater

Capitalize *greater* when referring to a specific community and its surrounding area. Lowercase otherwise.

> Greater Boston
> Greater Los Angeles
> the greater metropolitan area

See correspondence
  north, south, east, west
  Appendix J: American Cities and States

giga-

Prefix meaning *1 billion units of a measure.*

To convert to basic unit, move decimal point nine places to the right (adding zeros as necessary).

> 8.8 gigatons = 8,800,000,000 tons

globulins

Spell out English translations of Greek letters.

Place the arabic numeral (if included) on the line and connect it to the English translation of the Greek letter with a hyphen.

Use a character space before the word *globulin*.

> beta globulin
> beta-2 globulin

When using Greek letters, place a hyphen between the Greek letter (with or without subscript) and *globulin*.

> β-globulin
> β_2-globulin

Immunoglobulins are expressed as follows:

> IgA
> IgD
> IgE
> IgG
> IgM

gm

Alternative abbreviation for *gram*, but *g* is preferred.

Do not use a final period for either form.

> 4 g *preferred to* 4 gm

See gram

G

government

Always lowercase this term.

> federal government
> US government
> Canadian government
> taxes paid to the government

Capitalize full proper names of governmental agencies, departments, and offices.

> the US House of Representatives
> the US Supreme Court

Use capitals in shortened versions if the context makes the name of the nation, state, province, etc., clear.

> the House of Representatives
> Parliament

Lowercase the plural forms of terms such as *Senate* and *House of Representatives*, which are capitalized in proper names.

> California Senate and New York Senate
> *but* California and New York senates

gr

Abbreviation for *grain*. Do not confuse with *g* or *gm*, which are abbreviations for *gram*.

See grain

grade

Do not capitalize.

Use arabic numerals as a general rule, but check appropriate references for specific guidelines.

> grade 4 tumor

See cancer classifications
classification systems
orthopedics

grain
Smallest unit in US system of weights. Weight of one grain of wheat. There are 437.5 grains in an ounce, 7000 grains in a pound.

Abbreviation: *gr* (no period).

gram
Basic unit of weight in metric system. Approximately one twenty-eighth of an ounce.

Multiply by 0.035 to convert to ounces. *

Abbreviation: *g* is preferred to *gm* (not *gr*, which is the abbreviation for *grain*).

Gram stain
A method of differential staining of bacteria devised by Hans Gram, a Danish physician.

Capitalize the *G* in *Gram stain*.

> We ordered a Gram stain stat.

Lowercase *gram-negative* and *gram-positive*.

> The specimen was gram-negative.
> The culture grew out gram-positive cocci.

grammar

Correct the originator's obvious grammatical errors.

See dictation problems
    editing

grammar software

Software that automatically checks the grammar of a document. Grammar software is a supplement to, not a replacement for, the medical transcriptionist's responsibility to proofread documents and assure the accuracy of the grammar within them. Many grammatical errors will pass the scrutiny of software, and many acceptable choices will be unnecessarily questioned.

gray (Gy)

The International System unit of absorbed dose of ionizing radiation. Equal to 1 joule per kilogram of tissue.

Abbreviation: *Gy* (no period).

greater

The word *greater* is overused in medical parlance and is often dictated inappropriately when *more, longer,* or *over* would be a better choice of words.

As so often happens, shorthand is used in a handwritten patient chart, and a dictating physician will read the chart while dictating and will use the words that go with the shorthand symbol, when that may not be the best translation of the symbol. The symbol for *greater than (>)* is a part of the medical jargon that is particularly overused.

> D: The pain persisted greater than 24 hours.
> T: The pain persisted longer than 24 hours.

or The pain persisted more than 24 hours.

or The pain persisted over 24 hours.

See geographic names
greater than, less than (>, <)

greater than, less than (>, <)

The greater than and less than symbols are often mistaken for their opposite in meaning, and the Institute for Safe Medication Practices advises against their use.

> The patient's performance on the trial is in the impaired range (289 seconds, less than the 1st percentile).
> She weighed less than 100 pounds.
> The patient exhibited greater lung capacity following treatment.

Edit inappropriate uses of the expression *greater than* when another term (*longer than, more than,* or *over*) is more correct.

> D: He weighed greater than 300 pounds.
> T: He weighed over 300 pounds.

See Appendix B: Dangerous Abbreviations

Greek letters

Spell out the English translation when the word stands alone. Do not capitalize English translations.

Use the Greek letter or spell it out when it is part of an extended term, according to the preferred form; consult appropriate references for guidance.

> alpha   α
> beta   β
> gamma   γ

G

In extended terms, use of a hyphen after the Greek letter is optional, but the hyphen is not used after the English translation.

β-globulin *or* B globulin
beta globulin

GVHD grading system
See classification systems

H

h, h.

Letter *h* (without a period) is the abbreviation for the English word *hour*. Do not use except in virgule constructions and in tables.

> 40 mm/h
> The procedure lasted 1 hour 15 minutes.

Letter *h.* (with a period) is the abbreviation for the Latin word *hora*, meaning *hour*.

> q.6 h. (every 6 hours)

In instructions for medications, Latin abbreviations may be coupled with English terms, such as hour. These may be transcribed as dictated or the English translated to Latin.

> every 4 hours *or* q.4 hours *or* q.4 h *or* q.4 h.

See drug terminology

Health Care Financing Administration (HCFA)

See Centers for Medicare and Medicaid Services (CMS)

H

healthcare, health care

While some authors write *health care* as two words for every usage, AAMT's preference is that *healthcare* is written as one word when used as an adjective, two words *(health care)* when used as a noun.

> In order for this patient to receive proper health care, he should be seen on a monthly basis.

> This healthcare facility is not equipped to deal with these sorts of patients.

heart sounds and murmurs

See cardiology

hecto-

Inseparable prefix denoting *100 units of a measure.*

Use *hect-* before a vowel, *hecto-* before a consonant.

To convert to basic unit, move decimal point two places to the right, adding zeros as necessary.

> 3.3 hectometers = 330 meters

height

Express with numerals, as indicated below.

Write out nonmetric units of measure; do not use the symbols ″ and ′ for *inches* and *feet.*

Note: There is no comma between units of the same dimension, so there is no comma after *feet* in the following example:

> Height: 5 feet 8 inches.

Hemoccult

Hemoccult is a trade name and must be capitalized, even when used in a compound form.

>The exam was Hemoccult-negative.
>
>*or* The exam showed Hemoccult [test] was negative.

hepatitis nomenclature

Use capital letters to designate type.

Do not use a hyphen to connect the word *hepatitis* to the letter designating its type, but do use a hyphen to connect *non* to the letter.

>hepatitis A
>
>hepatitis C
>
>non-A hepatitis
>
>non-B hepatitis
>
>non-A, non-B hepatitis
>
>delta hepatitis

>### *related abbreviations*
>
>| | |
>|---|---|
>| HAV | hepatitis A virus |
>| HBAg | hepatitis B antigen |
>| HBsAg | hepatitis B surface antigen |
>| HBIG | hepatitis B immunoglobulin |
>| HBV | hepatitis B virus |
>| anti-HAV | antibody to hepatitis A |
>| anti-HBV | antibody to hepatitis B |

Previous designations of viral hepatitis, such as infectious hepatitis, short-incubation-period hepatitis, long-incubation-period hepatitis, and serum hepatitis are no longer preferred but should be transcribed if dictated.

H

hertz

International unit of frequency equivalent to one cycle per second.

Abbreviation: *Hz* (no period).

HIPAA

The Health Insurance Portability and Accountability Act of 1996 is legislation created to save costs by simplifying the administration of health care. Administered by the US Department of Health and Human Services, HIPAA includes regulations related to healthcare transactions and code sets, privacy of health information, security of information, and the establishment of national identifiers for providers and employers.

See confidentiality
   security

Hispanic

Adjective referring to a US citizen or resident of Latin American or Spanish descent. *Latina/Latino* are also widely used, and *Mexican American* or *Chicana/Chicano* may be preferred by those of Mexican descent. Transcribe as dictated.

See Chicana, Chicano
   Latina, Latino
   Mexican American
   sociocultural designations

historic periods and events

Capitalize widely recognized names for events in history, geology, archeology, anthropology, and for historic periods and events.

   the Middle Ages
   the Vietnam War

Capitalize only proper nouns and adjectives in generic descriptions of periods and events.

>   ancient Greece

Lowercase references to centuries.

>   20th century

history and physical examination

Abbreviation: *H&P* (no spaces, no periods). Typical major content headings in a history and physical, taken from ASTM's *E2184, Standard Specification for Healthcare Document Formats*, include the following:

>   CHIEF COMPLAINT
>   HISTORY OF PRESENT ILLNESS
>   PAST HISTORY
>   ALLERGIES
>   CURRENT MEDICATIONS
>   REVIEW OF SYSTEMS
>   PHYSICAL EXAMINATION
>   MENTAL STATUS EXAMINATION
>   DIAGNOSTIC STUDIES
>   DIAGNOSIS
>   ORDERS

See formats
>   Appendix A: Sample Reports

H

holidays and holy days

Capitalize the names of secular and religious holidays.

> Ascension Thursday
> Easter
> Fourth of July
> Kwanzaa
> Ramadan
> Rosh Hashanah

hopefully

Hopefully means *in a hopeful manner.*

> They waited hopefully for news of his recovery.

Strictly speaking, *hopefully* should not be used to mean *I hope, we hope, it is hoped, let us hope.* However, it is so widely used in this sense that such use is increasingly acceptable. Transcribe such usage if dictated.

> Hopefully, his symptoms will respond to the treatment.

hormones

Hormones may be referred to by their therapeutic or diagnostic names, their native names, or their abbreviations.

In abbreviated form, place numerals on the line or subscript.

therapeutic/diagnostic name	native name	abbreviation
chorionic gonadotropin	human chorionic gonadotropin	HCG
corticotropin, purified	corticotropin *(previously adrenocorticotropic hormone)*	ACTH
triiodothyronine	triiodothyronine	T3 *or* T_3
thyrotropin	thyroid-stimulating hormone	TSH
thyroxine	thyroxine	T4 *or* T_4

The preferred suffix is *-tropin* (indicating *an ability to change or redirect*), not *-trophic* (indicating *a relationship to nutrition*).

thyrotropin-releasing hormone
gonadotropin-releasing hormone
corticotropin
somatotropin

however

as an adverb

However may be used to modify one or more adjectives.

However resistant she may be, I will continue to advise her to quit smoking.

as a conjunctive adverb

Place a semicolon before and a comma after *however* when it is used to connect two complete, closely related thoughts in a single sentence.

He is improved; however, he cannot be released.

Place a comma after *however* when it serves as a bridge between two sentences.

> The patient was released from care. However, his wife called to say his condition had worsened again.

as an interruptive

When *however* occurs in the second sentence and is not the first word, it is called an interruptive and requires a comma before and after it. There is disagreement among grammarians as to the best placement of this type of *however*. In medical transcription, place it as dictated provided such placement does not interfere with communication.

> D&T: He is improved. He cannot, however, be released.
>
> D&T: He is improved. He cannot be released, however.

human leukocyte antigen (HLA)

Test that detects genetic markers on white blood cells. Abbreviation: *HLA*.

Express with capital-lowercase combinations and hyphens. Check appropriate references for guidance.

HLA-DR5	associated with Hashimoto thyroiditis
B8, Dw3	associated with Graves disease

major histocompatibility complex, class I antigens

> HLA-D
>
> HLA-DR

major histocompatibility complex, class II antigens

> HLA-B27
> HLA-DRw10

examples of antigenic specificities of major HLA loci

> HLA-A
> HLA-B
> HLA-C
> HLA-D

-hundreds

Numerals are preferred to words.

> 1900s *not* nineteen-hundreds

hyphens

Hyphens as word connectors or joiners may be permanent or temporary. Over time, hyphenated terms may be replaced with the solid form. Check appropriate English and medical dictionaries for guidance.

Do not space before or after a hyphen with the exception of suspensive hyphens (*See* suspensive hyphens *below*).

clarity

Use hyphens to avoid confusion in meaning.

> re-create (make again) *not* recreate (play)
> re-cover (cover again) *not* recover (from illness)
> re-place (put back in place) *not* replace (provide a substitute)

Use hyphens to assist in pronunciation.

> co-workers
>
> re-study

suspensive hyphens

Single-space after a suspensive hyphen (one used to connect a series of compound modifiers with the same base term).

> We used 3- and 4-inch bandages.

We do not recommend using what might be called a "suspensive" hyphen in an expression such as *intra- and extrahepatic ducts*; rather, we would write out both words in full: *intrahepatic and extrahepatic ducts*.

vowel strings

Sometimes, use a hyphen to break up a string of three or more vowels, but other times do not; again, a dictionary should be your guide.

> ileo-ascending
>
> *but* radioactive

missing letters or numbers

Use a double hyphen or dash to represent missing letters or numbers. Be sure to place a space after the double hyphen or dash used to represent the ending letters or numbers in a term.

> The patient said, "What the h— did he think I would do?"

telephone numbers

Use hyphens following the area code and prefix of a telephone number. Alternatively, the area code may be placed in parentheses. If an extension is given, it is common practice to label it *ext.*

209-555-9620, ext. 104

(209) 555-9620, ext. 104

ZIP codes

Use a hyphen between the first five and last four digits of a ZIP-plus-four code.

Modesto, CA 95354-0550

(Several more examples of hyphen usage follow. The rules that apply to these examples are found under a variety of headings throughout this book.)

adjectives

15-year-old boy

The patient is a 33-year-old.

2-year 5-month-old child

5½-year-old girl *or* 5-1/2-year-old girl

5 x 3 x 2-cm mass

The abdomen shows a 4-1/4-inch scar.

3- to 4-cm lesion

1-month course

.38-caliber pistol

two-thirds full

one-half normal saline

half-normal saline

Stool is heme-negative.

hyphens

She was panic-stricken

mucus-coated throat

20-pack-year history

self-medicated

shell-like

See compound modifiers

nouns

fracture-dislocation

son-in-law

ex-husband

helper-suppressor

numbers and letters

CIN-1 *or* CIN grade 1

ST-T segment

Q-wave pathology

3-0 suture material

beta-2 globulin

β-globulin
β2-globulin

non-A, non-B hepatitis

HLA-B27

C-section

2-D echo

Obstetric history: 4-2-2-4.
gravida 3, 3-0-0-3

C1-2 disk space

in place of dash

The patient agreed to return tomorrow—if he felt like it.

range

8-12 wbc

The office is open 1-4 p.m.

I

identical

Follow by *with* or *to*. Transcribe as dictated.

> The symptoms are identical with (*or* to) those he exhibited on his last admission.

inch

One twelfth of a foot. Metric equivalent: 2.54 centimeters. Multiply by 2.54 to convert to centimeters.

Write out; do not use abbreviation *(in.)* or symbol *(")* except in tables. When abbreviating *in.*, always use a period.

Express with numerals.

Do not use a comma or other punctuation between units of the same dimension, e.g., feet and inches.

> 12 feet 10 inches

incomparable words

Absolute adjectives that do not have a comparative or superlative form. They include *complete, dead, fatal, pregnant, total, unanimous,* and *unique.*

Forms such as *more complete* or *slightly pregnant* or *fatally dead* are inappropriate. Terms such as *almost* or *nearly* are, however, acceptable.

> almost fatal
> nearly total

initials

at end of transcript

See formats

in names

See personal names, nicknames, and initials

-in-law

Use hyphens.

> sister-in-law

Plural form: Make primary noun plural; do not add *s* to *law*.

> sisters-in-law

Possessive form: Use *'s* after *-law*.

> sister-in-law's
> sisters-in-law's

International System of Units (SI)

The International System of Units (Système International d'Unités, abbreviated SI) is the system of metric measurements adopted in 1960 at the Eleventh General Conference on Weights and Measures of the International Organization for Standards.

Since the 1977 recommendation of the 30th World Health Assembly that SI units be used in medicine, some medical journals use the SI to a limited degree, some use it only in conjunction with conventional units, and some have not yet adopted it.

The adoption of SI in the documentation of patient care is likewise sporadic, but it is sufficiently widespread, in whole or in part, to warrant the attention of medical transcriptionists. It should be noted that, although some units from the apothecary system remain in use, all elements of the apothecary system have been dropped from the compendium of the United States Pharmacopeia (USP) system.

Additionally, the accelerated movement toward international adoption of the electronic patient record is likely to strengthen the adoption of the SI in order to facilitate communication across borders.

Major characteristics of the SI are decimals, a system of prefixes, and a standard defined as an invariable physical measure.

basic units and properties of the SI

base unit	*SI symbol*	*basic property*
meter	m	length
kilogram	kg	mass
second	s	time
ampere	A	electric current
kelvin	K	thermodynamic temperature
candela	cd	luminous intensity
mole	mol	amount of substance

Two supplementary units of the SI are

radian	rad	plane angle
steradian	sr	solid angle

units derived from SI's basic units

derived unit	name and symbol	basic unit derived from
area	square meter (m^2)	meter
volume	cubic meter (m^3)	meter
frequency	hertz (Hz)	second
work, energy	joule (J)	kilogram
pressure	pascal (Pa)	kilogram
force	newton (N)	kilogram
density	kilogram per cubic meter (kg/m^3)	kilogram
speed, velocity	meter per second (m/s)	meter
acceleration	meter per second squared (m/s^2)	meter
electric field strength	volt per meter (V/m)	meter

prefixes and symbols

The SI combines prefixes with the basic units to express multiples and submultiples of those units. Factors are powers of 10. Note that the SI refers to shortened forms of measure as symbols, not abbreviations.

factor	prefix	symbol
10^{24}	yotta-	y
10^{21}	zetta-	z
10^{18}	exa-	E
10^{15}	peta-	P
10^{12}	tera-	T
10^9	giga-	G
10^6	mega-	M
10^3	kilo-	k
10^0	hecto-	h
10	deca-	da
10^{-1}	deci-	d

factor	prefix	symbol
10^{-2}	centi-	c
10^{-3}	milli-	m
10^{-6}	micro-	mc
10^{-9}	nano-	n
10^{-12}	pico-	p
10^{-15}	femto-	f
10^{-18}	atto-	a
10^{-21}	zepto-	Z
10^{-24}	yoctu-	Y

According to the *AMA Manual of Style*, exponents that are multiples of 3 are recommended, and those prefixes that are not multiples of 3 (e.g., *hecto-, deca-, deci-,* and *centi-*) are to be avoided in scientific writing. That avoidance obviously does not extend to patient records, as evidenced by MTs' frequent encounters with the prefix *centi-* (centimeter, centigrade, centigray) and occasional encounters with *deci-* (decigram, deciliter).

In general, medical transcriptionists should apply the following rules and guidelines for the SI, but this is not always possible. Exceptions that are necessary, logical, or commonly accepted in medical transcription are noted.

abbreviations

Abbreviate most units of measure that accompany numerals and include virgule constructions.

Use the same abbreviation for singular and plural forms.

Do not use periods with abbreviated units of measure.

1 g
20 g
40 mm/h

area, volume, and magnification

The SI uses the multiplication sign in expressions of area, volume, and magnification.

In medical transcription, use a lowercase *x* for area and volume; space before and after it to enhance readability.

> 2 x 2-mm area

Magnification is generally expressed with a capital *X* (although a lowercase *x* is acceptable), placed before the size of magnification, without a space.

> X30 magnification

commas

Drop the comma in numbers of four digits.

In numbers of five or more digits, the SI replaces the comma with a half space. This is not always possible in medical transcription, nor is it commonly seen in healthcare records, so the continued use of the comma is acceptable and preferred in numbers of five or more digits in medical transcription.

Do conform to the SI rule eliminating both the comma and the half space in numbers that contain decimal points.

> 1234
> 12,345
> 12345.67

decimals v fractions

Use the decimal form of numbers when a fraction is given with an abbreviated unit of measure or for a precise measurement.

Use mixed fractions for approximate measurements; these often represent time.

4.5 mm
5-1/2 days *or* 5½ days
3-3/4 hours

drug dosages

It is anticipated that all drug dosages will eventually be expressed in SI units.

See Appendix B: Dangerous Abbreviations

exponents

When technology does not readily allow exponents to be expressed as superscripts, abbreviations like *cu* and *sq* are acceptable.

Do not place the exponent numerals on the line in these expressions as they are not easily read when expressed in this manner.

10^5 *or* 10 to the 5th
3 m^2 *or* 3 sq m (*not* m2)
9 m^3 *or* 9 cu m (*not* m3)

kelvin v Celsius

The SI unit for thermodynamic temperature is the kelvin, but the medical transcriptionist is more apt to encounter temperatures reported in degrees Celsius or degrees Fahrenheit.

Transcribe the system dictated; do not convert.

numerals

Use arabic numerals for all quantities with units of measure.

Place a space between the numeral and the symbol for the unit of measure. Exceptions: Do not place a space between the numeral and the percent sign, the degree sign, or the Celsius (or Fahrenheit) symbol.

Place the quantity and the unit of measure on the same line of text; where possible, do not allow one line of text to end with the quantity and the next line to begin with the unit of measure.

> 48 kg
> 13.5 mm
> 48%
> 40°C

When a number and unit of measure begin a sentence, consider recasting the sentence so as to avoid beginning it with a numeral and unit of measure. Otherwise, write out both the number and unit of measure.

> D: Twenty milliequivalents of KCl was given.
> T: KCl 20 mEq was given.
> *or* Twenty milliequivalents of KCl was given.

percentage values

According to the SI, it is common and acceptable for percentage values to be expressed as a fraction of one. MT experience would indicate that it is more common and acceptable for *percent* to be dropped in dictation (and thus in transcription).

Use the expression dictated. Do not convert unless the forms are mixed; then make them consistent.

> polys 58% *or* polys 0.58 *or* polys 58
> MCHC 34% *or* MCHC 0.34 *or* MCHC 34

rad v gray; calorie v joule

The SI converts *rad* to *gray (Gy)* and *calorie* to *joule*.

Transcribe as dictated; do not make the conversion unless directed to do so.

units of time and time abbreviations

Do not abbreviate expressions of English units of time except in virgule constructions.

Do not use periods with such abbreviations.

Note: In pharmaceutical expressions such as *q.h.* and *q.i.d.*, the terms are Latin *(h., hora; d., die)* and require periods for clarity.

minute	min
week	wk
month	mo
hour	h
day	d
year	y

The patient is 5 days old.

He will return in 1 week for followup.

40 mm/h

q.4 h.

Efforts have been made here to extract the basic applications of SI rules and guidelines to medical transcription. As indicated, SI usage affects or is affected by many other areas of medical transcription style and practice: grammar, abbreviations, numerals, punctuation, plurals, etc.

More detail about the SI and SI units is available from the *AMA Manual of Style*, from which much of the above information was drawn, but keep in mind that the AMA text speaks to the preparation of medical manuscripts for publication and does not address the preparation of medical reports, i.e., the communication of patient information through medical dictation and transcription. As indicated, some of the differences are pronounced.

Note: For complete details of the Systèm International, visit the National Institute of Standards and Technology website at: http://physics.nist.gov/cuu/Units/.

See abbreviations, acronyms, brief forms
  drug terminology
  numbers
  Appendix B: Dangerous Abbreviations

Internet
See confidentiality
  correspondence
  security

intervertebral disk space
See orthopedics

italics
Italicized type is generally more difficult to read than regular type. Avoid its use in medical transcription, even with foreign words and phrases, genus and species names, or for emphasis.

When irony is intended, or for slang, coined expressions, inexact usage, or unusual usage where italics might generally be required, use quotation marks instead.

  an "impatient" patient
  rather than an *impatient* patient

For titles of books, periodicals, plays, films, long poems, paintings, sculptures, and legal case titles in text, use either italics or underlining.

> We refer to *The Surgical Word Book* often.
> *or* We refer to <u>The Surgical Word Book</u> often.
> *or* We refer to "The Surgical Word Book" often.

it's, its

Do not confuse or misuse these soundalikes.

it's

Contraction for *it is* and *it has*.

> It's time to go.
> It's been a long time since we saw this patient.

Remember that contractions are best avoided in healthcare records except in direct quotes.

its

Possessive form of *it*.

> Its dimensions were recorded by the nurse.

HINT: Italics and other attributes such as bolding or underlining may be lost in electronic transmission of reports, in which case quotation marks may be preferable.

J

Jaeger eye chart

Pronounced *yay-ger*. A *J* followed by an arabic numeral on the same line specifies the line with the smallest letters that the patient can read. Do not space between the letter and number.

J5

jargon

See language to avoid

JCAHO

Abbreviation for *Joint Commission on Accreditation of Healthcare Organizations*, an independent, not-for-profit organization that develops organizational standards, awards accreditation decisions, and provides education and consultation to healthcare organizations.

Jew

Use for both men and women; do not use *Jewess*. Adjective form: *Jewish*.

job descriptions

Do not confuse job descriptions with formal titles. Always lowercase job description namcs.

The patient is an administrative assistant in the surgery department.

Johns Hopkins University

Johns not *John* or *John's*.

joule

SI unit of energy. Pronounced *jewel*.

Plural is *joules*.

Abbreviation: *J* (no period).

The patient's atrial fibrillation was treated with the defibrillator set at 200 joules.

junior

Lowercase *junior* in references to academic class and member of class. Do not abbreviate *Jr.* unless used as part of a person's name.

She is a junior at Central High.
The junior class dance is tomorrow night.

Jr., Jr

See personal names, nicknames, and initials

K

K

abbreviation for Kelvin
See temperature, temperature scales

chemical symbol for potassium

KCl *(potassium chloride)*

thousand
Do not use *K* as an abbreviation for *thousand*.

$30,000 *not* $30K
platelets 340,000 *not* platelets 340K
WBC 12,000 *not* WBC 12K

Kelvin, kelvin
Capitalize when referring to the Kelvin temperature scale; lowercase when referring to a unit of temperature on that scale.

kilo-
Prefix meaning *1000 units of a measure.*

To convert to basic unit, move decimal point three places to the right, adding zeros as necessary.

11.8 kilograms = 11,800 grams

kilocycle
Another term for *kilohertz*.

Abbreviation: *kc* (no period).

kilogram
Metric term for 1000 grams (about 2.2 pounds or 35 ounces).

Abbreviation: *kg* (no period).

To convert to basic unit, move decimal point three places to the right, adding zeros as necessary.

$$11.8 \text{ kg} = 11,800 \text{ g}$$

To convert to pounds, multiply by 2.2.

$$2 \text{ kg} = 4.4 \text{ pounds}$$

kilohertz
Metric term for *1000 hertz* (1000 cycles per second); also known as *kilocycle*.

Abbreviation: *kHz* (no period).

kilometer
Metric term for *1000 meters*, approximately 3281 feet or 0.62 mile.

Abbreviation: *km* (no period).

To convert to basic unit, move decimal point three places to the right, adding zeros as necessary.

11.8 km = 11,800 m

To convert to miles, multiply by 0.62.

4 km = 2.48 miles

kind, kinds

Use *that* with *kind*, *those* or *these* with *kinds*. Watch subject-verb agreement.

That kind of lab value is ambiguous.
Those kinds of decisions are difficult.

K

L

L

Abbreviation for *liter*. The *L* is capitalized instead of lowercased so that it won't be mistaken for the number *1*.

lab

Short form for *laboratory*. Acceptable if dictated, except in headings and subheadings.

laboratory data and values

Use numerals to express laboratory values.

punctuation

Do not use commas to separate a lab value from the test it describes.

> white count 5300 *not* white count, 5300

When multiple lab results are given, separate related tests by commas. Use semicolons if entries in the series have internal commas.

> White count 5.9, hemoglobin 14.6, hematocrit 43.1.

Separate unrelated tests by periods. If uncertain whether tests are related or unrelated, use periods.

> White count 5.9, hemoglobin 14.6, hematocrit 43.1. Urine specific gravity 1.006, pH 6, negative dipstick.
>
> Blood work showed white count of 4800 with 58 segs, 7 bands, 24 lymphs, 8 monos, 2 eos, and 2 basos; hemoglobin 14.6 and hematocrit 43.1.

electrolytes

Substances that dissociate into positive and negative ions in solution. The electrolytes generally include sodium, potassium, chloride, and total CO_2 or bicarbonate. Anion gap may also be reported.

Though not technically electrolytes, BUN, creatinine, and glucose are also part of a chemistry profile and often dictated in the same breath.

> DIAGNOSTIC DATA
> Electrolytes: Sodium 139, potassium 4.6, chloride 106, bicarb 28.
> BUN 15, creatinine 0.9, glucose 132. White count 5.9,
> hemoglobin 14.6, hematocrit 43.1.

Gram, gram

Capitalize the *G* in *Gram stain*, but lowercase *gram-negative* and *gram-positive*.

> 3+ gram-positive cocci

hemoglobin and hematocrit

Hemoglobin and hematocrit values are often dictated "H and H" or "H over H." For clarity, translate the abbreviations into their respective terms.

> D: H and H 11.8 and 35.3.
> T: Hemoglobin 11.8 and hematocrit 35.3.

percentage values

Use the expression dictated.

> MCHC 34%
> *or* MCHC 0.34
> *or* MCHC 34
>
> polys 58%
> *or* polys 0.58
> *or* polys 58

Do not convert unless the forms are mixed; then make them consistent.

> D: White count was 4800 with 58 segs, 7 bands, 24 lymphs, 8 monos, 2% eos, and 2% basos.
> T: White count was 4800 with 58 segs, 7 bands, 24 lymphs, 8 monos, 2 eos, and 2 basos.

specific gravity
Express with four digits and a decimal point placed between the first and second digits.

Do not drop the final zero.

> D: specific gravity ten twenty
> T: specific gravity 1.020

tumor cell markers
Express with capital letters and arabic numerals, without spaces or punctuation between letter and number.

> CD4
> CD52

urinalysis
Term evolved from *urine analysis*, which is now archaic. Edit to *urinalysis*.

Use abbreviation *UA* only if dictated.

> D: Urine analysis showed...
> T: Urinalysis showed...

See blood counts
blood groups
globulins
human leukocyte antigen (HLA)
lymphocytes

L

language to avoid

Modern medicine is constantly evolving and so is its language. In addition, with the fast pace of American health care, clinicians sometimes find themselves dictating their notes on the fly, before they have had a chance to put their thoughts together. The result may be an awkward use of language and frequent neologisms (newly formed words).

Sometimes a noun or adjective is used as a verb. If possible, edit awkwardly created verbs.

> D: Stool was guaiac'd.
> T: Stool guaiac test was done.

Likewise, if possible, edit proper nouns dictated as verbs.

> D: The baby was de-lee'd on the abdomen.
> T: The baby was suctioned on the abdomen using DeLee.

back formation

New word formed by altering an existing word (usually a noun). Back formations are often verbs but may appear as adjectives or adverbs. They are frequently encountered in medical dictation. Use dictated back formations if they have become acceptable through widespread use. Avoid absurd back formations or ones that will be confusing to the reader.

original word	*back formation*
dehiscence	to dehisce
diagnosis	to diagnose
torsion	to torse

It is difficult to say which back formations will never become accepted; this is ultimately determined by usage. False verbs and other back formations are increasingly prevalent in the communications industry and technical world, but they should be used judiciously in transcribed health records, which are, after all, medicolegal documents that have a potentially long life.

coined terms

Non-official, non-standard terms. Many are back formations. Avoid as much as possible.

> We *lased* the tattoo in one session. (removed by laser)

jargon

Special language that is used and fully understood only by members of a particular craft, trade, or profession. Like other jargons, that of the healthcare professions parallels, but only slightly overlaps, formal technical terminology. It consists partly of lay and technical terms to which special meanings are assigned. It is largely unrecorded in reference books and is highly informal, including some expressions that are slangy or humorous. Medical jargon tends to be particularly imprecise and may be offensive or derogatory.

In general, avoid the use of jargon by rephrasing.

> D: urines
> T: urine samples

> D: FLK (*meaning* funny-looking kid)
> T: _____
> (leave blank and flag for alternative description)

slang

In general, avoid slang terms and phrases except when they are essential to the report, when they more accurately communicate the meaning than their translation would, or when their meaning cannot be determined.

dexamethasone *not* dex

appendectomy *not* appy

language to rewrite

The following examples illuminate the types of language that should be edited or left blank and flagged. Bring the usage of badly chosen dictated language that may be offensive to the attention of the appropriate person— e.g., supervisor, originator, service owner, client, risk manager—because they may create a risk management situation.

obscenities

Obscenities, profanities, and vulgarities do not belong in a patient's record unless they are part of direct quotations that are essential to the report.

derogatory or inflammatory remarks

In general, derogatory or inflammatory remarks do not belong in medical reports except in direct quotations, and then only when they are pertinent and essential.

double entendres

Double entendres are words or word combinations, as well as abbreviations and chemical symbols, that have varying meanings depending on context. Edit in order to avoid unintentional (and usually inappropriate) humor or derogatory implications.

D: He is complaining of some SOB.
T: He is complaining of some shortness of breath.

See dictation problems
    editing

languages
Capitalize the proper names of languages and their dialects.

The patient speaks Laotian and English.
Her Australian accent was difficult to understand.

laser
Acronym for **l**ight **a**mplification by **s**timulated **e**mission of **r**adiation, which through widespread use has evolved into a word in its own right and thus is not capitalized.

last, latest
Use *latest* instead of *last* unless finality is intended.

The latest white count showed...

Avoid *last* to indicate a particular month or day. Note: Don't guess at the date!

The patient was seen last Thursday, November 21, 2001.
not The patient was seen last Thursday.

Latin abbreviations
e.g., et al., etc., i.e., viz.
These Latin abbreviations are commonly used in English communications and need not be translated, although the medical transcriptionist should understand their meaning before using them.

The use of periods within or at the end of these Latin abbreviations remains the preferred style, although it is also acceptable to drop the periods.

abbreviation	Latin	English
e.g. *or* eg	exempli gratia	for example
et al. *or* et al	et alii	and others
etc. *or* etc	et cetera	and so forth
i.e. *or* ie	id est	that is
viz. *or* viz	videlicet	that is, namely

Use a comma **before and after** the abbreviation (or its English equivalent).

Her symptoms come on with exertion, e.g., when climbing stairs or running.
Her symptoms come on with exertion, for example, when climbing stairs or running.

She continued to be uncooperative, i.e., she refused all treatment.
She continued to be uncooperative, that is, she refused all treatment.

drug-related abbreviations
See drug terminology

See parenthetical expressions

Latina, Latino
Adjective referring to a US citizen or resident of Latin American or Spanish descent. Use *Latina* for a female, *Latino* for a male. Plural form is *Latinos*. *Hispanic* is also widely used, and *Mexican American* or *Chicana/Chicano* may be preferred by Americans of Mexican descent. Use whatever term is dictated.

See Chicana, Chicano
    Hispanic
    Mexican American
    sociocultural designations

lay, lie

These terms are easily confused because their meanings are similar and because the present tense of *lay* is also the past tense of *lie*.

lay

To place, to put, to deposit (something). It requires a direct object. Past tense and past participle *laid*, present participle *laying*.

> Please lay the book on the table.
> He laid the book on the table last week.
> He had laid the book on the table before the accident.
> He was laying the book on the table.

lie

Refers to a state of reclining. It does not take a direct object. Past tense *lay*, past participle *lain*, present participle *lying*.

> The patient was told to lie down and put her feet up.
> Her symptoms subside when she lies down.
> She lay on a gurney in the ER for 4 hours.
> She had lain down frequently.
> The patient was lying supine at the start of the procedure.

lead

verb

Past tense is *led* not *lead*.

> She led the AMA's delegation to the White House.

cardiac leads

See cardiology

length

Express with numerals.

> The scar was 4 inches in length.

lesbian

The preferred term to identify a homosexual woman. Lowercase except in names of organizations.

> *See* gay

less than (<)

See greater than, less than (>, <)

letters used as symbols

hyphens

Use a hyphen to join some compound nouns with a number or single letter as a prefix; in other instances, separate them by a space. Check appropriate references (i.e., dictionaries, word books) for specific terms.

> C-section
> x-ray
> R wave
> Z line

When an unhyphenated word of this type acts as an adjective preceding a noun it becomes hyphenated.

> T cell
> *but* T-cell count

plurals

Use *'s* to form the plural of single letters.

> p's and q's
> A's and B's

level

Position in a graded scale of values.

Lowercase *level* and use arabic or roman numerals according to the preferred style for the system being referenced.

> ***See*** cancer classifications
> classification systems
> orthopedics

like

preposition

In its prepositional form, *like* takes the objective case.

> She looks like me.

conjunction

Use *like* to introduce a noun that is not followed by a verb.

> He exercises *like* an athlete. *(not as an athlete)*

Use *as*, not *like*, to introduce a clause.

> He took the medication *as* he was instructed. *(not like he was instructed)*

HINT: When using *like* or *as* to make a comparison, remember that *like* is followed by a noun and *as* is followed by a clause.

lists

horizontal lists

There are two styles of horizontal lists, also called narrative or run-on. With both styles, enclose arabic numerals in parentheses to delineate the items in the list.

AAMT's preferred style is to use commas at the end of each item in a horizontal list. Use semicolons instead of commas if an item contains internal commas. Do not capitalize items separated by commas or semicolons.

> Her past history includes (1) diabetes mellitus, (2) cholecystitis, and (3) hiatal hernia.

> Her past history includes (1) diabetes mellitus, which is controlled with oral agents; (2) cholecystitis, resolved; and (3) hiatal hernia.

The other style choice is to use a capital letter to start each item in the list and use a period at the end of each item.

> Her past history includes (1) Diabetes mellitus. (2) Cholecystitis. (3) Hiatal hernia.

A colon may be used in place of the verb to introduce either type of list.

> Past history: (1) diabetes mellitus, (2) cholecystitis, (3) hiatal hernia.
> Past history: (1) Diabetes mellitus. (2) Cholecystitis. (3) Hiatal hernia.

vertical lists

For vertical (or *displayed*) lists, use block style, with all entries aligned at the left margin.

If numbered, follow each arabic numeral by a period and then one character space; do not place numbers in parentheses.

Capitalize the first letter of each entry, whether or not numbered (but it is preferable to number the items if there is more than one).

Place a period at the end of each entry in the list.

> 1. Diabetes mellitus.
> 2. Cholecystitis.
> 3. Hiatal hernia.

> FINAL DIAGNOSES
> Type 2 diabetes mellitus.
> Gastroenteritis.

If the entries in the list are names or dates, no period is used.

> SURGEONS
> Mabel Smith, MD
> Harry Jones, MD

hanging indentation

Alternative form for displayed lists. This style works best with display lists that are presented in sentence form.

Use arabic numerals.

L

Begin the first line of each item (the number) at the left margin and indent subsequent lines.

> ASSESSMENT AND PLAN
> 1. Hypertension. Blood pressures continue to run high. Will start the patient on Lotensin 20 mg p.o. daily, which may be increased to 40 mg next month if her numbers do not come down.
> 2. Diabetes. Continue the glyburide, which the patient is currently taking twice a day in divided doses. May consider reducing this if blood sugars stay within normal or if hypoglycemia becomes a problem. Continue the Actos begun last month.
> 3. Return in 4 weeks for followup. Patient instructed in recording blood pressure readings. She will also monitor her blood glucose twice a day.

See formats
> Appendix A: Sample Reports

liter

Basic unit of volume in the metric system. One liter is equal to the volume occupied by one kilogram of water at 4 degrees Celsius. One liter is also equal to 1000 cubic centimeters, 1000 milliliters, 34 fluidounces, 1.06 liquid quarts, or 0.91 dry quart.

Multiply by 1.06 to convert to liquid quarts.

Multiply by 0.91 to convert to dry quarts.

Multiply by 0.26 to convert to liquid gallons.

The abbreviation *L* is used instead of a lowercase *l*, which can easily be misread as the numeral *1* (one).

-ly

Do not use a hyphen between **adverbs** that end in *-ly* and the adjectives they modify.

> overly anxious parent

However, do use a hyphen between **adjectives** that end in *-ly* and the adjectives they modify.

> squirrelly-faced stuffed animal

See compound modifiers

lymphocytes

T lymphocytes (T cells) and B lymphocytes (B cells) are the most common lymphocytes.

T means *thymus-derived*, *B* means *bursa-derived*.

In general, do not use the extended forms.

hyphenation

Do not hyphenate except when used as an adjective preceding a noun.

> T cells
> T-cell count

pre- and pan-

Use a hyphen to join *pre-* or *pan-* to the following letter or word.

> pre-T cell
> pan-B lymphocyte
> pan-thymocyte

subsets of T lymphocytes

Use a virgule (not a hyphen) to express helper/inducer and cytotoxic/suppressor subsets of T lymphocytes.

> Helper/inducer T lymphocytes are also known as helper cells or helper T lymphocytes.
>
> Cytotoxic/suppressor T lymphocytes are also called suppressor cells.

Use a hyphen (not a virgule or colon) in the phrase *helper-suppressor ratio.*

> helper-suppressor ratio
>
> *not* helper/suppressor ratio
>
> *not* helper:suppressor ratio

surface antigens

Join arabic numerals (on the line) to the letter *T* to express surface antigens of T lymphocytes.

> T3
>
> T8
>
> T11

M

macro

A macro is a keyboard command that incorporates two or more other commands or actions.

Medical transcriptionists often use macros to reduce the number of keystrokes (and the amount of time) needed to transcribe frequently used phrases or paragraphs. Software programs that create macros are also called *abbreviation expanders* or *text expanders*.

Beware of creating macros that are words in their own right, or you may make mistakes similar to the following:

> Dear Paroxysmal Atrial Tachycardia (*when* Dear Pat *was intended*)
> Liver and spleen Vegas (*when* Las Vegas *was intended*)

macro-

A prefix meaning *extra large* or *long*.

Join the prefix directly to the term that follows, without hyphenation. The usual exceptions for prefixes apply.

> macroaggregate
> macrocephaly

magnification
X

Magnification is generally expressed with a capital X (although a lowercase x is acceptable) placed before the size of magnification, without a space.

X30 magnification

loupe magnification

A loupe is a magnifying lens. *Loop* is **not** an acceptable alternative.

main clause

See clauses

margins

See formats

master's degree

Lowercase as a general rule. Capitalize only when it follows a person's name.

Joan Shafer, Master of Education

See degrees, academic
Appendix I: Professional Credits and Academic Degrees

MD

Abbreviation for *Doctor of Medicine.*

Preferred style is without periods. If periods are used, do not space within the abbreviation (M.D., *not* M. D.).

Set off the abbreviation by commas.

Mary Smith, MD, was called in for consultation.

mean, median

The *mean* is the average of a group of numbers.

The median is the number at the midway point in a series of numbers listed in ascending or descending order.

> Exam scores were 48, 49, 53, 88, and 92.
> The mean score on the exam was 66.
> The median score on the exam was 53.

media

Plural of *medium*, so it takes a plural verb.

> The contrast media were...

The term *optic media* refers to all the different substances in the eye through which light travels. Therefore, a plural verb is required.

> The optic media were...

medical language specialist

An alternative (descriptive) title for medical transcriptionist.

Do not capitalize; do not abbreviate.

> Rhonda Williams, medical language specialist

See certified medical transcriptionist (CMT)
   credentials, professional
   Appendix C: Medical Transcription Job Descriptions

M

medical specialties

Do not capitalize the names of medical specialties or their variations that designate the practitioners of those specialties. These are common nouns, not proper nouns.

> The orthopedist's evaluation...
> Her specialty is cardiology.
> The surgeon was Dr. Doolittle.

medical transcription

The process of interpreting oral dictation by physicians and other healthcare professionals and recording the content in a written form (whether print or electronic), while editing simultaneously to produce a grammatically correct document. The dictation is commonly related to patient assessment, workup, diagnostic and therapeutic procedures, treatment and clinical course, prognosis, and patient instructions. The resulting document is the record of patient care that is necessary to facilitate delivery of healthcare services.

The process of medical transcription may involve editing machine-translated text. This involves listening to dictation while reading a draft created through speech recognition technology and editing the text on screen. This editing may range from minimal to extensive, depending on the capabilities of the speech recognition software and the dictating habits of the originator, and may include correction of content as well as punctuation, grammar, and style.

See Appendix C: Medical Transcriptionist Job Descriptions

mega-

Prefix meaning *1 million units of a measure.* To convert to basic unit, move decimal point six places to the right, adding zeros as necessary.

Join *mega* to its root word without a hyphen.

> 3.8 megatons = 3,800,000 tons

mEq

Abbreviation for *milliequivalent*.

Use with numerals.

Do not use periods.

Do not add *s* for plural.

Space between the numeral and the unit of measure.

> 20 mEq

meridians

Imaginary location lines that circle a globular structure, such as the eye, at right angles to its equator and touching both poles. Measured in units of 0 degrees to 180 degrees.

> The eye was entered at the 160-degree meridian.

In acupuncture, meridians connect different anatomic sites.

meter

Basic unit of length in the metric system. Equal to 39.37 inches, usually rounded to 39.5 inches.

To convert to inches, multiply by 39.37. To convert to yards, multiply by 1.1.

Abbreviation: *m* (no period).

metric system

See International System of Units
units of measure

M

Mexican American

Designates an American of Mexican descent. More widely preferred than *Chicana/Chicano*. Transcribe whatever term is dictated. Do not hyphenate.

See Chicana, Chicano
Latina, Latino
Hispanic
sociocultural designations

mg

Abbreviation for *milligram*.

Do not use periods.

Do not add *s* for plural.

Space between the numeral and the abbreviation.

>   5 mg

Do not use fractions with metric units of measure.

>   5.5 mg *not* 5½ mg

mg%

Abbreviation for *milligrams percent*. Equivalent to milligrams per deciliter (mg/dL), which is the preferred nomenclature, but transcribe as dictated.

Do not use periods.

Do not add a space between *mg* and *%*.

Do add a space between the numeral and *mg*.

    23 mg%

micro-

Prefix meaning *one-millionth of a unit*. Use the abbreviation *mc*. (The *mu* sign [μ] should not be used as it is often misread and is on the list of "Dangerous Abbreviations and Dose Designations" [**See** Appendix B: Dangerous Abbreviations].)

To convert to basic unit, move decimal point six places to the left.

    14,596 mcg = 0.014596 g

When spelling the word in full, the prefix *micro-* is usually joined directly to the term that follows, i.e., without hyphenation. The usual exceptions for prefixes apply.

    micromanage
    microscopy

See Appendix B: Dangerous Abbreviations

mid, mid-

Can stand alone or serve as a prefix.

When used as a prefix, *mid* is usually connected to the word element without a hyphen, but there are the usual exceptions.

    midabdominal mass   midpalmar crease
    midday   mid and distal palmar creases
    midlung field   mid-Atlantic
    right midlung   mid-90s
    mid to lower lung fields

Middle East
Capitalize as indicated. Adjective form: *Middle Eastern.*

midnight
Technically, the end of a day, not the beginning of a new one, so it is equivalent to 12 p.m.

Do not capitalize. Do not use *12* with it.

> Twin A was born at midnight, December 31, 2001; twin B at 12:14 a.m., January 1, 2002.

Midwest, Middle West
Capitalize as indicated.

Adjective forms: *Midwestern, Middle Western.*

mile
Equal to 5280 feet or 1609 meters.

Multiply by 1.6 to convert to kilometers.

Do not abbreviate.

Express with numerals.

> 14 miles = 22.4 km

Use the abbreviation *mph* or *MPH* for *miles per hour* (either form is acceptable) only when preceded by numerals.

Do not use periods.

> 84 mph
> *or* 84 MPH

military terminology

military units

Use arabic ordinals and capitalize key words when expressed with figures.

> The 2nd Infantry Division...

Capitalize *company* only when it is part of a name; do not abbreviate it.

> Company C *not* Co. C

military time

See time

military titles

See titles

milli-

Prefix meaning *one-thousandth of a unit.*

To convert to basic unit, move decimal three places to the left.

> 1384 mg = 1.384 g

milliequivalent (mEq)

One-thousandth equivalent, i.e., the number of grams of a solute that are contained in one milliliter of a one normal (1N) solution.

Abbreviation: *mEq* (no periods; note the capital *E*).

20 mEq

milligram (mg)

One-thousandth of a gram. Equals approximately 1/28,000 of an ounce.

To convert to ounces, multiply by 0.000035.

Abbreviation: *mg* (no period).

milliliter (mL)

Unit of liquid measure. One-thousandth of a liter. Equal to approximately one-fifth of a teaspoon.

To convert to teaspoons, multiply by 0.2. One fluidounce equals 30 mL.

Abbreviation: *mL* (no period).

millimeter (mm)

One-thousandth of a meter. Approximately 0.04 inch.

To convert to inches, multiply by 0.04. One centimeter equals 10 mm.

Abbreviation: *mm* (no period).

millisecond (ms or msec)

One thousandth of a second.

Abbreviation: *msec* (no periods).

M

minus, minus sign (-)

Write out the word *minus* if you are not certain the symbol will be noticeable or clear.

> minus 40

Write out *minus* to indicate below-zero temperatures.

> minus 38 degrees *not* -38 degrees

If you do use the sign, express with a hyphen, not a dash; do not space between the hyphen and numeral.

> -40

Plus or minus or *plus/minus* should be spelled out in full and not expressed as *+/-* or ± except in tables.

Miss

Courtesy title for a woman or girl. Plural form is *Misses*.

> The Misses Brown, White, and Green...

The preferred form for a woman or girl is *Ms*, but use the term dictated.

See titles

mL

Abbreviation for *milliliter*. The abbreviation *mL* is preferred to *ml* to avoid the *l* being misread as the numeral *1 (one)*.

Use with numerals.

Space between the numeral and the unit of measure.

Do not use periods.

Do not add *s* for plural.

50 mL

Do not use fractions with metric units of measure.

2.5 mL *not* 2½ mL

mm

Abbreviation for *millimeter*, unit of measure for length, breadth, width, depth, height, etc.

Use with numerals.

Space between the numeral and the unit of measure.

Do not use periods.

Do not add *s* for plural.

50 mm

Do not use fractions with metric units of measure.

7.25 mm *not* 7¼ mm

M

mmHg

Abbreviation for *millimeters of mercury*. Use with pressure readings (blood pressure, tourniquet pressure, etc.). Need not use if not dictated.

Do not use periods.

> D: BP 110/90
> T: BP 110/90 mmHg
> *or* BP 110/90

It is also acceptable, but not preferred, to space between *mm* and *Hg*: *mm Hg*.

months

Capitalize the names of months.

Do not abbreviate except in tables and in military style, and even then, do not abbreviate *March, April, May, June, July,* unless all of the months are expressed as three-letter abbreviations without ending periods.

month	*standard abbreviation*	*3-letter designation*
January	Jan.	Jan
February	Feb.	Feb
March	March	Mar
April	April	Apr
May	May	May
June	June	Jun
July	July	Jul
August	Aug.	Aug
September	Sept.	Sep
October	Oct.	Oct
November	Nov.	Nov
December	Dec.	Dec

M

Mount, Mt.

Abbreviate or spell out in proper names according to common or preferred usage related to entity in question.

> Mount Vernon
> Mt. Shasta

Spell out and lowercase generic uses.

> The patient was injured while climbing a mountain.

mph, MPH

Abbreviation for *miles per hour*. Either form is acceptable, though using all capitals places unnecessary emphasis on the units of measure.

Do not use periods.

Do not add *s* for plural.

Space between the numeral and the abbreviation.

> 40 mph
> *or* 40 MPH

Mr., Mr

Abbreviation for *Mister*. Courtesy title for a man. It may be expressed with or without the ending period.

Plural: *Messrs.*

See titles

Mrs., Mrs

Courtesy title for a married or widowed woman. May be written without the ending period.

Plural: *Mmes.*

See titles

Ms, Ms.

Courtesy title for a woman or girl. Preferred over *Miss.* Since *Ms* is not an abbreviation, it is usually written without the ending period. There is no plural form; repeat *Ms* before each name.

Ms Brown, Ms Green, and Ms White

See titles

msec, ms

Abbreviations for *millisecond.* Do not use periods.

Do not add *s* for plural.

Space between the numeral and the abbreviation.

280 msec

MT

Abbreviation for *medical transcription* and for *medical transcriptionist* (also for *medical technologist, music therapist, massage therapist).*

No periods.

Plural: *MTs.*

Possessive: *MT's* (singular) or *MTs'* (plural).

Do not use *MT* following a name because doing so gives it the appearance of being a recognized professional credential, which it is not. The only recognized professional credential for medical transcriptionists is CMT (certified medical transcriptionist).

> Rhonda Williams, medical transcriptionist
> *not* Rhonda Williams, MT

See certified medical transcriptionist (CMT)
> credentials, professional
> Appendix C: Medical Transcriptionist Job Descriptions

mucus, mucous

Mucus is the noun form.

> She coughed up mucus.
> Mucus-type tissue was noted. (*Use the noun form with* -type.)
> The wound is mucus-producing. (Mucus *is the object of the present participle verb, so the noun form, not the adjective form, must be used.*)

Mucous is the adjective form.

> mucous membrane
> The mucous discharge is of concern.

Avoid the word *mucosy*. Edit to *mucous* or *mucus-like*.

> D: There was a mucosy texture to the discharge.
> T: There was a mucus-like texture to the discharge.

multiplication symbol
See X, x

murmurs, cardiac
See cardiology

M

N

namely

Latin equivalent is *videlicet,* abbreviated *viz.*

Place a comma both before and after *viz.*

> The patient refused to follow medical advice, viz., take her medication.

See Latin abbreviations

names

confidentiality

AAMT advises against the use of a patient's name in the body of a medical report. In fact, any data that may lead to the identification of a specific patient should be limited to the demographic section of the report. In this way, if the report is ever used for scientific study or any other reason, personal information can be readily deleted from it.

See confidentiality

proper name

Specific name of a person, place, or thing.

Capitalize most proper names. (Occasional exceptions exist, based on the individual's personal preference, e.g., e.e. cummings.)

> the White House

Do not use an apostrophe in plural forms of proper names.

The Smiths were referred by...
All Toms, Dicks, and Marys were there.

proprietary product names

The brand name is the manufacturer's name for a product; it is the same as the trademark or proprietary name.

Capitalize the initial letter of the trademark or brand name of drugs, sutures, instruments, etc. In the case of oddities such as pHisoHex, where there is eccentric use of capitals, it is acceptable to either (1) match the manufacturer's presentation or (2) use initial capital only. However, when the manufacturer uses all capitals, use an initial capital only so as not to give undue attention to the term in a medical report.

It is not necessary to use the trademark symbols (^{TM} or $^{®}$) in patient care documents.

Do not capitalize adjectives and common nouns associated with trademark or brand names.

examples of brand names or trademarks
Diprolene cream
RhoGAM *or* Rhogam
Ligaclip (*not* LIGACLIP [the manufacturer's style])
intravenous Valium
Adaptic gauze dressing
running Dacron sutures
Hemoccult test

The trade name is a broader term than trademark, identifying the manufacturer but not the product. Capitalize trade names; again, do not use all capitals even if the manufacturer does.

examples of trade names
Bayer

Dr. Scholl's

generic product names
A generic name is an established, nonproprietary name for a drug, suture, instrument, etc. Its use is unrestricted. Do not capitalize generic names; they are common nouns.

examples of generic names
aspirin

catgut sutures

imipramine

milk of magnesia

nomenclatures
Numerous nomenclatures, or naming systems, are used in medicine to promote the consistent, correct, and stable naming of entities; only selected ones are addressed in this style book.

AAMT guidelines for expressing nomenclatures in transcription take into account recommendations and guidelines from reliable sources, e.g., the *AMA Manual of Style* and the American Diabetes Association. We have also considered technological capabilities and deficiencies (for example, in relation to subscripts and superscripts) in order to promote consistency, ease of use, and communication. Thus, acceptable forms in medical transcription may differ from official forms, as well as from forms within manuscripts.

nano-
Prefix meaning *one-billionth of a unit.*

To convert to basic unit, move decimal point nine places to the left.

4987870984.4 nanoseconds = 4.9878709844 seconds

nation, national

Lowercase except when part of a proper name or formal title.

The Fourth of July is a national holiday.
"Face the Nation" is a television program.

nationalities

Capitalize proper names of nationalities, peoples, races, tribes, etc.

British
Sioux

Hyphens are generally not used when describing Americans by their nationality of origin.

African American
French Canadian

Do not use derogatory or inflammatory terms associated with nationalities except in direct quotes that are essential to the report. Bring inappropriate usage to the attention of those responsible for risk management.

negative findings

Negative findings are those within normal limits; they are also referred to as normal findings. Positive findings are those not within normal limits.

Negative or normal findings may be as important to diagnosis and treatment as are positive or abnormal findings. Recording such findings provides medicolegal documentation that the related tests or exams were done and were normal and reduces the unnecessary repetition of tests or procedures to determine findings, in turn reducing healthcare costs.

Transcribe all findings dictated, whether identified as positive, negative, or normal.

negative sign (-)

Do not use except in tables or special applications, e.g., blood nomenclature. Also avoid if its usage may cause the reader to overlook it.

> blood type O negative
> *preferred to* blood type O-

no one, none

no one

Takes a singular verb.

> No one expects him to recover full use of the arm.

none

May be singular *(not one, no one, no single one)* or plural *(no two, no amount, not any)*, taking singular or plural verbs and pronouns as appropriate.

> We tried to identify the bleeding site; none was found. *(not one site was found)*
> We found 4 bleeding sites; none were cauterized. *(no sites were cauterized)*

Use context to determine if singular or plural form is intended. If either could be used, assume it is singular and use singular verbs and pronouns.

In the phrase *none of,* the object of the preposition *of* determines whether construction is singular or plural.

> None of *the findings are* conclusive.
> None of *it makes* sense.

nonmetric units of measure

See units of measure

noon

The middle of the day and end of the morning, equivalent to 12 a.m.

Lowercase.

Do not use *12* in conjunction with it.

> The infant was born at noon, January 14, 2001.

normal findings

Transcribe all dictation, even if referred to as *normal* or *negative* findings.

See negative findings

normal saline

Normal saline means *physiologic saline*—having the same concentration of sodium chloride (NaCl) and the same osmotic activity as intercellular fluid. Normal saline is 0.9% NaCl solution. Half-normal saline is a 1:2 dilution of normal saline, that is, 0.45% NaCl.

Express normal saline solutions as follows, as dictated.

> normal saline
> half-normal saline
> one-half normal saline
> quarter-normal saline

A mixture of dextrose and saline may be written as follows:

> D5 in half-normal saline *(5% dextrose in a solution of 0.45% sodium chloride)*

As a cautionary note: Solutions in general are expressed in terms of concentration, such as normality and molarity. Normal is expressed in gram-equivalents of solute per liter of solution, as follows: 0.5N (half-normal), 2N (twice normal).

Intravenous solutions are almost always administered as mass-produced, ready-to-infuse products. However, pharmacists have occasionally misinterpreted the phrase "normal saline" as 1N sodium chloride solution in making up ad hoc IV solutions, with serious consequences. A 1N sodium chloride solution contains 1000 mEq/L, hence about six times the concentration of normal (physiologic) saline.

Therefore, **do NOT use** 0.5N or N/2 for half-normal saline.

north, south, east, west (and their variations)
compass points and directions
Lowercase the term when referring to compass points or directions.

> Their house faces south.
> They headed east from California.
> They proceeded in a northerly direction.

N

geographic regions

Capitalize the term when it is part of a proper name of a state, country, region, or location.

> East Germany
>
> Northern Hemisphere
>
> South Carolina
>
> South Korea
>
> South Pole

Capitalize the term when referring to US coastal regions, but lowercase it when referring to the shoreline itself. (Use *the Coast* for references to the West Coast only.)

> He is from the East Coast.
>
> Some areas of the east coast have had severe storm damage.
>
> She returned to the Coast by air, landing in Los Angeles.

Capitalize the term when referring to geographic regions of the United States or when referring to a widely recognized region within a state, but lowercase it when referring to a less commonly recognized region within a state.

> She is from the Southwest.
>
> She is from Northern California.
>
> He is from northern New Hampshire.
>
> He is from the Midwest but has lived in the East for 20 years.
>
> She exaggerates her Southern accent.

Capitalize the term when referring to a native or resident of a geographic region of the United States.

> Louis L'Amour wrote classic novels about Westerners.

Capitalize the term when it is part of a phrase that is commonly used in reference to a city's section, but lowercase it if it is not a common designation.

> She grew up on Chicago's South Side.
> He lives on the south side of town.

Capitalize *Northwest* in reference to that territorial section of Canada.

> Northwest Territories

Capitalize *West/Western* when referring to the Occident, *East/Eastern* when referring to the Orient.

> Western dress is increasingly common in Eastern countries.

ideological divisions

Capitalize *East/Eastern* and *West/Western* when referring to ideological divisions of the world.

> He was born in what was then an Eastern bloc country.

time zones

Some references capitalize the first word used in reference to a time zone, but some do not. Be consistent. (Note: *Pacific* should always be capitalized.)

> Eastern time zone *or* eastern time zone
> Mountain standard time *or* mountain standard time

nouns

Proper nouns name specific persons, places, and things. All other nouns are common nouns. It may help to think of proper nouns as brand names and common nouns as generic terms. Do not capitalize common nouns in an attempt to give them the stature of proper nouns.

> He was admitted to *St. Mary's Hospital. (proper noun)*
> She was seen in the *emergency room* of St. Mary's Hospital. *(common noun)*

Nouns usually are subjects or objects of a sentence. Sometimes, they may be modifiers.

> She became ill while attending an *educators* conference. (*not* educators' conference)

Use the possessive form for a noun or pronoun that precedes a gerund (verb ending in *-ing* and used as a noun).

> *His dieting* is a problem.
> The *patient's screaming* disturbed other patients.

Use the possessive form for a noun involving time, measurement, or money that is used as a possessive adjective.

> The pain was of 3 months' duration.

collective noun

Represents a collection of persons or things regarded as a unit.

Usage determines whether the collective noun is singular or plural. It is singular and takes a singular verb when the total group it represents is emphasized. It is plural and takes a plural verb when the individuals making up the group are emphasized.

examples of collective nouns

board (of directors)	majority
class	number
committee	pair
couple	set
family	staff
group	team

The group is meeting frequently throughout its stay.

The group of patients were female. *(each was female)*

A number of adhesions were present. (*individual adhesions were present, not a collective adhesion*)

The number of adhesions was minimal. (*The subject* the number of *always takes a singular verb.*)

The couple were injured in a plane crash.

but The couple has an appointment with the geneticist.

Treat units of measure as singular collective nouns that take singular verbs.

At 8:30 this morning, 20 mEq of KCl was administered.

noun-verb agreement

See subject-verb agreement

n.p.o.

See drug terminology

HINT:

A number = plural
(nonspecific)

The number = singular
(specific)

number of

A collective noun that may be singular or plural. If preceded by *the*, it takes a singular verb. If preceded by *a*, it takes a plural verb.

> *The* number of adhesions *was* minimal.
> *A* number of adhesions *were* present.

Use *number* to refer to persons or things that can be counted. *Number* tells how many; *amount* tells how much (mass).

> There was a small amount of bleeding, given the large number of wounds.

> A large number of people were present.
> *not* A large amount of people were present.

See amount of

numbers

Numerals, or figures, stand out from the surrounding text and serve a functional purpose in medical reports, where they should be used almost exclusively as opposed to spelled-out numbers.

> She was seen in the emergency room 1 hour after the accident.
> He tried 3 different medications without success.
> The specimen weighed less than 2 pounds.

exceptions

There are always exceptions to any rule, and judgment and discretion are needed when deciding whether to use numerals or spell out numbers.

adjacent numbers

When two numbers are consecutive, spell out one of them to avoid confusion.

> The patient was instructed to drink eight 8-ounce glasses of GoLYTELY before bedtime.
>
> Discharge Medication: Os-Cal 500 one daily.
>
> two 8-inch drains

Use a comma to separate adjacent unrelated numerals if neither can be readily expressed in words and the sentence cannot be readily reworded.

> In March 2002, 2038 patients were seen in the emergency room.

fractions

Spell out or use numerals for common fractions. Use the dictation style as a guide.

> An hour and a half before presentation, the patient slipped and fell.
>
> *or* Approximately 1-1/2 hours before presentation... (*if dictated "one and a half hours" or "one and one-half hours"*)
>
> The glass was two-thirds full. *or* The glass was 2/3 full.
>
> 7/8-inch wound
>
> a half-inch incision *or* a ½-inch incision (*since it was dictated precisely*)
>
> about a half inch below the sternal notch (*the word* about *makes this an imprecise measurement*)
>
> He smokes a pack and a half of cigarettes per day.
>
> *or* He smokes 1½ packs of cigarettes per day.
>
> *or* He smokes 1-1/2 packs of cigarettes per day.

N

beginning of a sentence

Spell out numbers that begin a sentence, or recast the sentence.

> D: Fourteen days ago she started having severe cramping.
> T: Fourteen days ago she started having severe cramping.
> *or* She started having severe cramping 14 days ago.

> **An exception to this exception:** A complete year that begins a sentence need not be spelled out.

> 2005 will mark our hospital's 100th anniversary.

> **Note:** Although it's acceptable to begin a sentence with a year, it is better to recast the sentence if possible.

> D: 1995 was when her symptoms began.
> T: Her symptoms began in 1995.

zero

Zero is always spelled out when it stands alone.

> The patient had zero response to the treatment.
> Her symptoms usually appear when the outside temperature drops below zero.
> *but*
> gravida 1, para 0
> 0°F

HINT: The "pronoun exception" applies if you can replace the number with another word that is not a number. The "one" in this example can be replaced by "x-ray," so *one* meets the test for the pronoun exception.

pronouns

Spell out numbers used as pronouns.

> The radiologist compared the previous x-rays with the most recent one.

numbers commonly spelled out

Common or accepted usage may dictate that a word be spelled out. For example, use of a numeral may cause confusion by placing emphasis and implying a precise quantity where none is intended.

> His symptoms went from one extreme to the other.
>
> The patient was given a choice between two courses of treatment; she chose the diet and exercise over medication.

nonspecific numbers

Spell out nonspecific (indefinite) numeric expressions.

> She described hundreds of symptoms. *(not 100s)*
>
> Several thousand people were tested.

arabic v roman numerals

There is a trend away from the use of roman numerals and toward the use of arabic numerals. A good example of this is in diabetes terminology, where an international expert committee dropped the roman numerals in favor of arabic, noting the danger of a roman numeral *II* being misread as an arabic number *11*. In addition, the *AMA Manual of Style* states, "Avoid the use of roman numerals except when part of established nomenclature."

arabic numerals

The arabic numerals are 0, 1, 2, 3, 4, 5, 6, 7, 8, 9.

Most numerals used in medicine are expressed as arabic numerals. Therefore, a general rule is to use arabic numerals unless roman numerals are specified or unless there is strong documentation that the preferred form is roman.

N

Grades are generally written in arabic numerals

> grade 3/6 holosystolic murmur
> CIN grade 3
> grade 3 chondromalacia patellae

See roman numerals *below, as well as* cancer classifications, classification systems, *and* orthopedics.

roman numerals

Do not use periods with roman numerals. Seven letters make up the roman numeral system. Capital letters are used except in special circumstances; e.g., lowercase letters (i, v, x, etc.) are used as page numbers for preliminary material (contents pages, preface, etc.) in a book.

> I = 1
> V= 5
> X = 10
> L = 50
> C = 100
> D = 500
> M = 1000

When a letter follows a letter of greater value, it increases the value of the preceding letter.

> VI   (5 + 1 = 6)

When a letter precedes a letter of greater value it diminishes the value of the following letter.

> IV   (5 - 1 = 4)

A bar over a letter indicates multiplication by 1000.

$$\overline{X} = 10,000$$

(Following are some common applications that use roman numerals. To determine arabic or roman numeral usage for other applications, check the arabic section of this topic and several other entries throughout this book, as well as other appropriate references [especially word books in the medical specialty involved].)

Stages are generally expressed with roman numerals, although there are exceptions.

> stage IV decubitus ulcer
> ovarian carcinoma, FIGO stage II
> stage 3 Garden fracture of femoral neck

cranial nerves
Arabic or roman numerals may be used.

> cranial nerves 1-12 *or* cranial nerves I-XII

wars, people, animals
Roman numerals are generally used for wars, people, and animals.

> World War II
> Henry Ford III
> Rover II
> *but* C. Roy Post 4th *(the personal preference of this cereal magnate)*

ordinals
Ordinal numbers are used to indicate order or position in a series rather than quantity.

N

Ordinals are commonly spelled out, especially when the series goes no higher than 10 items. However, as with all numbers in medical reports, AAMT recommends using numerals: 1st, 2nd, 3rd, 4th, etc.

Do not use a period with ordinal numbers.

> 3rd rib (*or* third)
> 5th finger (*or* fifth)
> She is to return for her 3rd (*or* third) visit in 2 days.
> She was in her 9th (*or* ninth) month of pregnancy.
> His return visits are scheduled for the 15th and 25th of next month.
> The 4th cranial nerve...

punctuation
hyphens
Use hyphens when numbers are used with words as compound modifiers preceding nouns.

> 5-cm incision
> 3 x 2-cm mass
> 13-year 2-month-old girl

Use hyphens to join some compound nouns with numbers as prefixes. Check appropriate references for specific terms.

> 2-D

Use hyphens in compound numbers from 21 to 99 when they are written out. (Note: The only time they should be written out is at the beginning of a sentence.)

> thirty-four
> one hundred fifty-three

commas

Use a comma to separate groups of three numerals in numbers of 5 digits or more, but omit the commas if decimals are used. The comma in 4-digit numerals may be omitted.

> Platelet count was 354,000.
> White count was 7100. *or* ...7,100.
> 12345.67

Do not place commas between words expressing a number.

> four hundred forty-eight
> *not* four hundred, forty-eight

plurals

Use *'s* to form the plural of single-digit numerals.

> 4 x 4's

Add *s* without an apostrophe to form the plural of multiple-digit numbers, including years.

> She is in her 20s.
> She was born in the 1940s.

multiple digits

When dictated in a form such as "four point two thousand" or "five point eight million," numerals may be transcribed in one of two ways:

> 4.2 thousand
> *or* 4200

> 5.8 million
> *or* 5,800,000

proper names

Use words or figures for numbers in proper names, according to the entity's preference.

> 20th Century Insurance
> Three Dollar Cafe

at end of line

When possible, do not separate numerals from the terms they accompany. Do not allow a numeral to end on one line and its accompanying term to begin the next.

> ....grade 2.
> *not*
> ....grade
> 2.

No.,

Abbreviation and symbol for *number*. Note that the abbreviation capitalizes the initial letter and has an ending period: *No.* When the symbol *#* is used, the numeral follows it with no space between.

> No. 4 blade
> #4 blade

position or rank

Use the abbreviation or symbol with a figure to indicate position or rank.

> He is No. 4 on the appointment list.
> *or* He is #4 on the appointment list.

model and serial numbers
Use the symbol with arabic numerals.

model #8546

serial #185043

sizes of instruments or sutures
Do not use the abbreviation or symbol if "number" is not dictated. Either is acceptable (with the symbol preferred to the abbreviation) if "number" is dictated. Be consistent.

5-French catheter, #5-French catheter, No. 5-French catheter

3-0 Vicryl, #3-0 Vicryl, No. 3-0 Vicryl

street addresses
Do not use the abbreviation or symbol before the number in street addresses.

166 Wallingford Avenue

not No. 166 Wallingford Avenue

not #166 Wallingford Avenue

suites, apartments, rooms
Use the abbreviation or symbol in suite, apartment, room, or similar number designations, when the noun designation is not used.

#104 *or* No. 104 *or* Apt. 104 *not* Apt. #104

schools, fire companies, lodges
Do not use the abbreviation or symbol in names of schools, fire companies, lodges, or similar numbered units.

Public School 4

Engine Company 3

numbers

(Examples of number usage appear under a variety of headings throughout this book. Several are mentioned here as well.)

ages

7-year-old child
15 years 3 months old

alphanumeric terms

G6PD
L4-5

clock referents

The lesion was seen in the left breast at the 8 o'clock position.
The incision was made from the 7:30 to 9:30 position.

decade references

The patient's father is in his 80s.
The patient hasn't been to a dentist since the '80s.

decimals

Cortrosyn 0.25 mg
.22-caliber rifle

EKG leads

V1 through V6
leads I, II, and III

eponyms

Apgar scores were 9 and 9.

Clark level II melanoma

Billroth II anastomosis

Hunt and Hess neurological grade 3

LeFort I maxillary reconstruction

O

obstetrics
abort, abortion
Transcribe this term as dictated (editing only as necessary for grammar and clarity). Although the *AMA Manual of Style* prefers the term *terminate* to *abort*, AAMT does not recommend making this editorial change if "abort" is dictated.

> D: abort
> T: abort (*not* terminate)

The abbreviations *AB* for *abortion*, *SAB* for *spontaneous abortion (miscarriage)*, and *TAB* for *therapeutic abortion* are often used as well.

GPA system
GPA is abbreviation for *gravida, para, abortus*. Accompanied by arabic numerals, *G, P*, and *A* (or *Ab*) describe the patient's obstetric history.

Use arabic numerals. Roman numerals are not appropriate.

G	gravida (number of pregnancies)
P	para (number of births of viable offspring)
A *or* Ab	abortus (abortions)

nulligravida	gravida 0	no pregnancies
primigravida	gravida 1, G1	1 pregnancy
secundigravida	gravida 2, G2	2 pregnancies
nullipara	para 0	no deliveries of viable offspring

Separate GPA sections by commas. Either the abbreviated or the spelled-out form may be used, whichever is dictated.

> Obstetric history: G4, P3, A1.
> *or* Obstetric history: gravida 4, para 3, abortus 1.

TPAL system

System used to describe obstetric history of a patient.

T	term infants
P	premature infants
A	abortions
L	living children

Separate TPAL numbers by hyphens.

> Obstetric history: 4-2-2-4.

TPAL numbers need not be spelled out unless dictated that way, for example

> Obstetric history: 4 term infants, 2 premature infants, 2 abortions, 4 living children.

Sometimes, GPA terminology is combined with TPAL terminology.

> The patient is gravida 3, 3-0-0-3.
> *or* gravida 3, para 3-0-0-3
> *or* G3, P3-0-0-3
> *or* gravida 3-0-0-3

cesarean section

Not *Cesarean, caesarean,* or *Caesarean.*

Brief form is *C-section*, but do not use it unless it is dictated, and even then do not use it in the operative title section of operative reports or discharge summaries.

fundal height

Distance from symphysis pubis to dome (top) of uterus. Expressed in centimeters.

After the 12th week of pregnancy, the number of centimeters should equal the number of weeks of pregnancy. If the measurement is larger, it may indicate large-for-dates fetus or multiple fetuses.

> Fundal height is 28 cm.

station

Term designating the location of the presenting fetal part in the birth canal. Expressed as -5 to +5, representing the number of centimeters below or above an imaginary plane through the ischial spines (station 0 is at the plane).

cervical cytology, Pap smear

See cancer classifications

ocean

Capitalize only when part of a proper name. Lowercase other uses.

> Pacific Ocean
> Arctic Ocean
> He became ill while on an ocean cruise.
> The Pacific and Atlantic oceans...

OD

Abbreviation for *oculus dexter*, meaning *right eye*, and for *Doctor of Optometry* degree. In either usage, capitalize and do not use periods.

Note that *o.d.* should not be used as an abbreviation for *every day*. Spell out *every day* or *daily* instead. This is on the list of dangerous abbreviations from the Institute for Safe Medication Practices.

See Appendix B: Dangerous Abbreviations

 off
Preposition. Do not follow by *of*.

> He fell off the roof.
> *not* He fell off of the roof

 oh
Do not capitalize except at beginning of sentence. Do not use *O* instead.

 only
Take care to place *only* next to the word it is modifying, or its meaning may be confused and impair clear communication.

> He is only able to walk 1 block. *(could be interpreted to mean he was only able to walk, not jog or run)*
> He is able to walk only 1 block. *(this clearly indicates the patient's limited ability to walk)*

 operate, operate on
A surgeon operates *on* a patient, and a patient is operated *on*. Add *on* even if not dictated.

> D: The patient was operated without incident.
> T: The patient was operated on without incident.

operative report

Typical content headings in an operative report include

preoperative diagnosis

postoperative diagnosis

reason for operation *or* indications

operation performed *or* name of operation

surgeon

assistants

anesthesiologist

anesthesia

indications for procedure

findings

procedure *or* technique

complications

tourniquet time

hardware

drains

specimens

estimated blood loss

instrument and sponge counts

disposition of patient

followup

See formats

Appendix A: Sample Reports

O

oral

In reference to language, *oral* refers only to words that are spoken. *Verbal* refers to words used in any manner, e.g., spoken, written, typed, printed, signed.

In reference to drug terminology, *oral* medications are taken by mouth.

ordinal numbers

See numbers

originator

One who originates the document in question, whether it be a report, letter, manuscript, etc., and whether it is dictated, handwritten, or dictated and automatically transcribed by a speech recognition engine. *Originator* is the preferred term, but *dictator* (in the case of dictation) or *author* may also be used.

originator's style

The transcriptionist is responsible for retaining the originator's style when translating the spoken word to text. Yet, the MT must also edit to assure the record's completeness, correctness, coherence, clarity, and readability. There is a fine line between appropriate editing, which the transcriptionist must do, and tampering, which the transcriptionist must diligently avoid.

See dictation problems
    editing
    language to avoid

orthopedics
  angles

In expressing angles, write out *degrees* or use the degree sign (°).

The patient was able to straight leg raise to 40 degrees.
or ...to 40°.

Catterall hip score

Rating system for Legg-Perthes disease (pediatric avascular necrosis of the femoral head).

Use roman numerals I (no findings) through IV (involvement of entire femoral head).

Crowe classification

System for classifying developmental dysplasia of the hip.

grade I	less than 50% subluxation
grade II	50% to 75% subluxation
grade III	75% to 100% subluxation

fracture classification systems

Garden

Subcapital fractures of femoral neck.

Lowercase *stage* and use arabic numerals: stage 1 (incomplete) through stage 3 (most complete).

LeFort

Classification of facial fractures.

Use roman numeral I, II, or III. Do not space between *Le* and *Fort*.

LeFort I

FOR ORthopedics in general use Roman Numerals per NAN

Mayo

Classification of olecranon fractures. Use roman numerals and capital letters.

type	description
I	undisplaced
IA	noncomminuted
IB	comminuted
II	displaced, stable
IIA	noncomminuted
IIB	comminuted
III	displaced, unstable
IIIA	noncomminuted
IIIB	comminuted

Neer-Horowitz

Classification of proximal humeral physeal fractures in children.

Use roman numerals I (less than 5-mm displacement) through IV (displaced more than two-thirds the width of the shaft).

Neer-Horowitz II

Salter

Classification of epiphyseal fractures.

Use roman numerals I (least severe) through VI (most severe).

Salter III fracture

Salter-Harris

Fracture involving the physis in children.

Use roman numerals I (fracture across the physis only) through V (crush injury to physis).

Salter-Harris fracture type II.

Schatzker

Classification of tibial plateau fractures in terms of injury and therapeutic requirements.

Lowercase *type* and use roman numerals: type I (least complicated) through type VI (most complicated).

stress fractures

Lowercase *grade* and use roman numerals I (local symptoms, negative radiographs, positive bone scan) through IV (local symptoms, actual bone fracture identified on radiographs, positive bone scan).

Note: A grade 0 indicates an asymptomatic patient with negative radiographs and negative bone scan.

Neer staging

System for classifying shoulder impingement.

stage	description
I	inflammation and edema of the rotator cuff
II	degenerative fibrosis
III	partial or full thickness tear

Outerbridge scale
Assesses damage in chondromalacia patellae.

Lowercase *grade*. Use arabic numerals 1 (minimal) through 4 (excessive).

> Diagnosis: Chondromalacia patellae, grade 3.

pins, screws, wires
Orthopedic pins, screws, and wires are generally measured in portions of an inch.

> D: a three thirty two Steinmann pin
> T: a 3/32-inch Steinmann pin

Kirschner wires are measured in portions of an inch but written using decimals.

> D: a four five K wire and a six two K wire
> T: a 0.45 K wire and a 0.62 K wire

vertebra
Expressed by a capital *C, T, L,* or *S* to indicate the region (*cervical, thoracic, lumbar,* or *sacral*), followed by an arabic numeral placed on the line (do not subscript or superscript). *D* for *dorsal* is sometimes substituted for *T (thoracic)*.

Do not use a hyphen between the letter and the number of a specific vertebra.

Do not subscript or superscript the numerals.

Plural: *vertebrae*.

> S1 *not* S-1
> T2 *or* D2

It is preferable to repeat the letter before each numbered vertebra in a list.

> The lesion involves C4, C5, and C6.
> *not* ...C4, 5, and 6.
> *and not* ...C4, 5, 6.

intervertebral disk space

Use a hyphen to express the space between two vertebrae (the intervertebral space). It is not necessary to repeat the same letter before the second vertebra, but it may be transcribed if dictated.

> C1-2 *or* C1-C2
> L5-S1

OS

Abbreviation for *oculus sinister, left eye.*

Capitalize.

Do not use periods.

ounce

Equal to 28 grams. To convert to grams, multiply by 28.

> 2 ounces = 56 grams

Write out; do not use abbreviation (*oz.*, with a period) except in tables.

Express accompanying numbers as numerals.

Do not use a comma or other punctuation between units for pounds and units for ounces.

The infant weighed 13 pounds 2 ounces.

fluidounce, fluid ounce

Either form is acceptable if dictated. The apothecary ounce equals 8 dr., 31.10349 g, 2 tablespoons, 6 teaspoons. Metric equivalent of a fluidounce (unit of volume) is approximately 30 mL, so to convert to milliliters, multiply by 30.

4 fluidounces = 120 mL

outlines

Use for displayed (vertical) lists with two or more values and levels, alternating numerals and letters. Each level should have two or more entries.

Use a period after divisional numerals and letters that are not in parentheses; do not use periods following numerals and letters that are in parentheses.

two-level outline

1.
   a.
   b.
2.

three-level outline

1.
   a.
   b.
     (1)
     (2)
2.

four-level outline

I.
    A.
    B.
       1.
       2.
          a.
          b.
II.

more than four levels

Repeat sublevels, placing numerals and letters in parentheses.

decimal outline form

1
    1.1
       1.1.1
       1.1.2
    1.2
    1.3

over

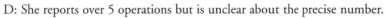

more than

When *over* means *more than*, replace it with *more than*.

> D: She reports over 5 operations but is unclear about the precise number.
>
> T: She reports more than 5 operations but is unclear about the precise number.

When *over* may mean *more than* or *for a period of* and you can determine the intended meaning, replace *over* with the more precise term.

> D: The rash persisted over 2 weeks.
>
> T: The rash persisted for over 2 weeks.
>
> *or* The rash persisted over a 2-week period.

If you cannot determine the meaning, transcribe as dictated and flag for the originator to clarify.

The rash persisted over 2 weeks.

virgule

Use a virgule to express *over* or *on a scale of* in expressions such as the following.

D: blood pressure 160 over 100
T: blood pressure 160/100

The following examples may be dictated with the words *over* or *out of* or *on a scale of.*

D: reflexes 2+ on a scale of 4
T: reflexes 2+/4

D: grade one over four murmur
T: grade 1/4 murmur

D: grade two to three over six murmur
T: grade 2/6 to 3/6 murmur
or grade 2 to 3 over 6 murmur

P

pacemaker codes

See cardiology

pack-year history of smoking

Smoking history expressed as an amount equal to packs smoked per day times number of years smoking.

Use numerals and hyphens as follows:

20-pack-year smoking history

In the above example, the patient's smoking history is equivalent to one pack per day for 20 years or two packs per day for 10 years or five packs per day for 4 years, etc.

page numbers

Lowercase *page* and use arabic numerals.

His history is detailed on page 2 of the report dated January 4, 2001.

Lowercase roman numerals (i, v, x, etc.) refer to page numbers for preliminary material (contents pages, preface, etc.) in a book.

Pap smear

The brief form for *Papanicolaou* is *Pap*, which may be used if dictated. If the full word is dictated, transcribe in full.

See cancer classifications.

para-, peri-

Speakers of American English don't always clearly distinguish the prefix *para-* *(next to)* from *peri-* *(around)*, partly because they often don't know or don't observe the differences in meaning. An originator may unconsciously, or even consciously, slur the pronunciation to cover his or her own uncertainty, perhaps hoping that the medical transcriptionist will resolve the ambiguity and transcribe the word correctly.

Word pairs such as *perifollicular* and *parafollicular*, many of which occur in the medical language, are practically homonyms, and the context of the dictation often gives no help in deciding between them. Pararenal fat is anatomically distinct from perirenal fat, yet either or both may be mentioned in the operative report of a nephrectomy. Some other word pairs (*paraumbilical* and *periumbilical*) are practically synonyms.

The transcriptionist who has a thorough grasp of medical terminology should have no trouble with terms such as *parasite, parathyroid, peristalsis*, and *peritoneum*. Other phrases such as *perihilar infiltrate, periorbital ecchymosis, paracolic gutter*, and *paranasal sinuses* occur so often that we have become familiar with them.

The semantic difference between *para-* and *peri-* is not clearly marked or consistently observed. However, there are certain patterns that can help decide which prefix is correct. Abstract nouns denoting diseases or conditions, particularly those ending in *-ia* or *-osis*, are more likely to begin with *para-* (paraplegia, parakeratosis). Terms for chemical substances begin with *para-* (parachlorophenol, parathion). Nouns denoting anatomic structures, particularly those ending in *-eum* or *-ium*, usually begin with *peri-* (pericardium, peritoneum). (Exception: parametrium.)

Adjectives denoting anatomic planes or lines and those referring to incisions generally begin with *para-* (parasagittal, paramedian). In official anatomic terminology, adjectives referring to lymph nodes begin with *para-* rather than *peri-* (parasternal, paratracheal). (Exception: pericardial lymph nodes, where the adjective means "draining the pericardium" rather than "around the heart.")

P

The difference in meaning between *para-articular calcifications* and *periarticular calcifications*, or between *para-appendiceal abscess* and *periappendiceal abscess* is so slight that most originators would be hard-pressed to say which adjective fits better or to find fault with the transcriptionist's choice.

parallel construction

Elements of a series should be parallel, e.g., nouns with nouns, gerunds with gerunds. Edit appropriately.

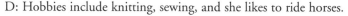

> D: Hobbies include knitting, sewing, and she likes to ride horses.
> T: Hobbies include knitting, sewing, and riding horses.

An unparallel series is also known as *bastard enumeration*.

With correlative conjunctions (either...or, neither...nor, not only...but also, both...and), use parallel construction on either side of the coordinating conjunction.

> D: She has both pain and she has fever.
> T: She has both pain and fever.

See conjunctions

parentheses ( )

Parentheses are used to provide parenthetical (incidental or supplementary) information that is not closely related to the rest of the sentence. They may or may not be dictated.

Use parentheses sparingly. If the parenthetical information is closely related to the rest of the sentence, use commas instead.

> A great deal of swelling was present, more so on the left than the right.
> *not* A great deal of swelling was present (more so on the left than the right).

brackets [ ]

Brackets may be used around a parenthetical insertion within a parenthetical insertion. Follow the rules for parentheses.

> The patient had had multiple complaints (headache, nausea, vomiting, and [he thought] fever) and demanded to be seen immediately.

Note: An originator will often dictate "brackets" instead of "parentheses" in error.

See chemical nomenclature *for the special placement of brackets in chemical and mathematical formulas.*

braces { }

Braces are used in chemical and mathematical formulas. (Note that the placement of parentheses and brackets is different in chemical and mathematical formulas than it is in regular text.)

> The chemical formula for hydroxychloroquine sulfate is 7-chloro-4-{4-[ethyl(2-hydroxyethyl)amino]-1-methylbutylamino}-quinoline sulfate.

See chemical nomenclature

capitalization

If the parenthetical entry is within a sentence, begin it with a lowercase letter and omit closing punctuation whether or not it is a complete sentence.

> Further past history shows outpatient pulmonary function tests with a forced vital capacity of 2.57 liters (equal to 62% of predicted) and an FEV of 0.98 liters.

A parenthetical entry that stands on its own (is not simply a part of a sentence) must be a complete sentence; start it with a capital letter and end it with closing punctuation inside the closing parenthesis.

Pelvic ultrasound was read as intrauterine changes consistent with pyometra. (It is difficult to believe that this diagnosis could be made on the basis of an ultrasound.)

commas

Do not precede either an opening parenthesis or a closing parenthesis by a comma.

Place a comma that follows the parenthetical information after the closing parenthesis mark.

> The patient is improving (despite her repeated insistence that she is dying), and we plan to discharge her to an extended care facility next week.

enumerated items within a sentence

Use arabic numerals within parentheses to enumerate items within a sentence.

Separate the enumerated entries by commas or semicolons.

> He has a long history of known diagnoses, including (1) chronic silicosis, (2) status post left thoracotomy, (3) arteriosclerotic cardiovascular disease.

parenthetical expressions

Expressions that interrupt the flow of the sentence.

Set off parenthetical expressions by commas (not parentheses, as one would expect by their name).

The commas may be omitted if their absence will not confuse the reader. In the following example, the parenthetical expressions appear in italics.

> A great deal of swelling was present, *more so on the left than on the right*. Ultimately this cleared, *however*, and azotemia too was reversed. It is *therefore* advisable that the patient continue bed rest.

Use a comma before and after Latin abbreviations (and their translations), such as *etc., i.e., e.g., et al., viz.*, when they are used as parenthetical expressions within a sentence.

We asked the patient to continue his regular medications, i.e., Actos and Lotensin.

pc, p.c.

Abbreviation *pc* is for *photocopy*, and *p.c.* is for *post cibum (after food)*.

per

See virgule

percent (%)

Note that *percent* is a single word.

Do not use the abbreviation *pct.* except in tables. Instead, use % or *percent*.

50% *or* fifty percent *not* 50 pct.

Use the symbol % after a numeral. Do not space between the numeral and the symbol.

13% monos, 1% bands
She has had a 10% increase in weight since her last visit.
MCHC 34%
10% solution

Use numerals for the number preceding %.

50% *not* fifty %

When the number is written out, as at the beginning of a sentence, write out *percent*.

Fifty percent of the patients were given a placebo.

According to the SI (International System of Units), it is common and acceptable for percents to be expressed as a fraction of one. MT experience would indicate that it is more common and acceptable for *percent* to be dropped in dictation (and thus in transcription). Use the expression dictated; do not convert.

> polys 58% *or* polys 0.58 *or* polys 58
> MCHC 34% *or* MCHC 0.34 *or* MCHC 34

range

In a range of values, repeat % (or *percent*) with each quantity.

> Values ranged from 13% to 18%.
> *not* Values ranged from 13 to 18%.

> Fifty percent to eighty percent...
> *not* Fifty to eighty percent...

subject-verb agreement

Percent of takes a singular verb when the word following *of* is singular, a plural verb when the word following *of* is plural.

Ninety percent of the body was burned.
Forty percent of the patients were in the control group.

Percent takes a singular verb when it stands alone (not followed by *of*).

> Fifty percent is adequate.

See subject-verb agreement

less than 1 percent

When the amount is less than 1 percent, place a zero before the decimal.

> 0.5% *not* .5%

With whole numbers, avoid following the number by a decimal point and a zero, since such forms are easily misread. The decimal point and zero may be used if it is important to express exactness. Use it if dictated.

5% *not* 5.0%

Use decimals, not fractions, with percents.

0.5% *not* 1/2%

percentage point

Percentage point is not the same as *percent*. Thus, a decrease from 10 percent to 5 percent is a decrease of 5 percentage points. It represents a decrease of 50 percent, not a decrease of 5 percent.

percentile

Probability distribution. If a boy's height is at the "50th percentile," he is at the same height as 50% of boys his age.

See International System of Units
range

periods

Periods are most commonly used to mark closure. They may also be used as a mark of separation.

Place a period at the end of a declarative sentence.

The patient's past medical history is unremarkable.

Place a period at the end of an imperative sentence that does not require emphasis. For emphasis, use an exclamation point.

Do not lift heavy objects.

Never lift heavy objects!

with other punctuation

Do not use a period at the end of a parenthetical sentence within another sentence.

> When I saw him on his return visit (Dr. Smith saw him on his initial visit), I was startled by the deterioration in his condition.

If a sentence terminates with an abbreviation (or other word) that ends with a period, do not add another period to end the sentence.

> He takes Valium 5 mg q.a.m.
>
> *not* He takes Valium 5 mg q.a.m..

Always place the period inside quotation marks.

> The patient's response was emphatic: "I will never consent to the operation."

in laboratory data

Separate values of unrelated tests by periods.

> White count 5.9. Urine specific gravity 1.006.

personal names, nicknames, and initials

Capitalize personal names.

> Stanley Livingstone

foreign names of persons

Follow the person's preference for spelling, capitalization, and spacing.

P

Capitalize or lowercase the foreign particles *de, du, di, d', le, la, l', van, von, ter,* etc., according to the preference of the individual named. Check appropriate references for guidance. Use lowercase if unable to determine preference. When a lowercase particle begins a sentence, it must be capitalized.

> De Pezzer catheters were used.
> *but* We inserted a de Pezzer catheter.

> a DeBakey procedure

initials

Use a period after each initial within a name (whether or not the initial stands for something), but do not use periods when initials replace a complete name.

> Harry S. Truman
> John F. Kennedy *but* JFK *not* J.F.K.

When an individual uses initials for first and middle names, do not space between them.

> T.S. Eliot

Do not use a single initial with a last name unless it is the person's preference or you cannot determine the first name.

> W. Madison

Jr., Jr; Sr., Sr

Abbreviations for *junior* and *senior* in names.

Usage of a comma before and a period after is optional, but use both or neither.

Do not use all capitals (JR, SR).

> Dr. Martin Luther King, Jr.
> *or* Dr. Martin Luther King Jr

nicknames

Do not use a nickname as the formal patient identifier unless the full name is not known. Otherwise, do not shorten a name or use a nickname unless that is the individual's clear preference. Do not enclose nicknames in quotation marks.

> Patricia Smith *as formal patient identifier, but otherwise* Pat Smith

ordinals

Do not place a comma after a name and before an ordinal. The ordinal may be roman or arabic; follow the preferences of the named individuals.

> John D. Rockefeller III

personifications

Capitalize personifications, such as Mother Nature.

> He kept saying, "You can't fool Mother Nature."

> We called Pathology and they reported a negative reading on the specimen.

words derived from eponymic or personal names

Do not capitalize words derived from eponymic or personal names.

> parkinsonism
> cushingoid
> cesarean

pH

Measure of acidity or alkalinity of a solution (e.g., urine or blood), ranging from 0 to 14, with 7 being neutral.

Express by a whole number or a whole number followed by a decimal point and one or two digits. A whole number may be followed by a decimal point and 0 to demonstrate that the value following the decimal point has not been mistakenly deleted.

> pH 7.55
> pH 7.4
> pH 7.0

Do not express other than with a lowercase *p* and capital *H*. If the term begins a sentence, precede it by *The* or recast the sentence.

> D: pH was 6.47.
> T: The pH was 6.47.

phase

Lowercase *phase* and use arabic numerals.

> phase 4

phrases

A phrase is a group of words without a subject or a verb, or both. It often begins with an adverb, preposition, or participle.

Use a comma before and/or after a phrase when the sentence could be misread without it, but do not use such commas if they change the intended meaning. Follow the guidelines below.

A comma following a short opening adverbial phrase is optional. Use the comma for longer introductory phrases or when its absence might cause confusion.

> *Presently* she is without pain.
> *Because of vomiting,* an NG tube was put in place.

An introductory prepositional phrase is always correct with a comma following it; it may also be correct without one. Never omit the comma if it is needed for clarity.

> *During hospitalization,* she will have a CAT scan.
> *During hospitalization* she will have a CAT scan.

Introductory expressions in which the subject and verb are understood are clauses, not phrases, and should always be followed by a comma.

> *After surgery,* he was taken to the recovery room.
> *If so,* he will return sooner. (If so *is understood to mean* if that is so.)

Do not use a comma before or after other prepositional phrases unless it is needed for clarity.

> The patient will return to my office *for continuing pain.*
> The exam revealed a young girl *with multiple injuries.*

Do not use commas to set off essential participial phrases. Use commas to set off nonessential participial phrases.

> Examination revealed 2 wounds *bleeding profusely* and several small bleeders.
> The incision, *running from the umbilicus to the symphysis pubis,* was closed in layers.
> The patient was admitted *screaming with pain.*

When a transitional phrase or independent comment occurs at the beginning of a second independent clause and it is preceded by a comma and *and, but, for, or, nor, yet,* or *so,* follow the transitional phrase with a comma.

> He was improving, but in spite of physical therapy, he still had difficulty walking without assistance.

Phrases such as *in addition to, along with, as well as, together with,* and similar terms are not conjunctions, and they do not create a compound subject. So, they do not change a singular verb to a plural verb. Watch usage.

> D: The patient, as well as his wife, were resistant to discussing alternative forms of treatment.
> T: The patient, as well as his wife, was resistant to discussing alternative forms of treatment.

Note: Replacing such a phrase with *and* would create a compound subject. Delete the commas and use a plural verb. (It is not appropriate, however, for an MT to make such a replacement.)

> The patient and his wife were resistant to discussing alternative forms of treatment.

See clauses
conjunctions

pico-

An inseparable prefix meaning *one-trillionth of a unit.*

To convert to the basic unit, move the decimal point 12 places to the left.

> 5,678,123,456,891.4 picoseconds = 5.678123456891 seconds.

pint

dry pint

Equal to 33.6 cubic inches (one-half of a dry quart). Its metric equivalent is 0.55 liter.

To convert to liters, multiply by 0.55.

liquid pint

Equal to 16 fluidounces or two cups. Its metric equivalent is 473 mL or 0.473 liter.

To convert to liters, multiply by 0.473.

plain film x-rays

Indicates that the x-ray was done without contrast. Not a CT scan, just a plain x-ray. Not *plane*.

Plain film of the abdomen was negative.

plane

An imaginary flat surface.

Planes of the body and its structures include those listed below. Check appropriate references (anatomy books and medical dictionaries) for additional planes.

frontal	a vertical plane dividing the body or structure into anterior and posterior portions. Also known as *coronal plane*.
sagittal	lengthwise vertical plane dividing the body or structure into right and left portions; midsagittal plane divides the body into right and left halves. Also known as *median plane*.
transverse	plane running across the body parallel to the ground, dividing the body or structure into upper and lower portions. Also known as *horizontal* or *axial plane*.

plant names

Capitalize the first word in a botanical name.

Lowercase other names of plants except the proper names or adjectives that are part of them.

Gardenia brighamii
Her favorite flower is gardenia, but she is allergic to it.

See genus and species names

plurals

Use the general rules to form plurals unless the dictionary provides the plural form. When the dictionary lists more than one plural form, the first is usually the preferred one.

gases *preferred to* gasses

In general, do not use apostrophes to form plurals, but there are exceptions.

abbreviations

Use 's to form the plural of lowercase abbreviations, but no apostrophe following all-capital abbreviations.

rbc's *not* rbcs *or* RBC's
WBCs
EEGs
PVCs

To form the plural of brief forms, add *s* without an apostrophe.

exams

segs

polys

differential diagnosis

When a patient presents with a group of symptoms and the diagnosis is unclear, the clinician may refer in the medical report to the *differential diagnosis* in order to compare and contrast the clinical findings of each. Although it consists of two or more possible diagnoses, the term *differential diagnosis* itself is singular and always takes a singular verb.

The differential diagnosis was...

letters, symbols

Use *'s* to form the plural of single letters and symbols.

serial 7's

names (including eponyms)

Add *s* (or *es*) without an apostrophe to form the plural.

Babinskis were positive.

The Joneses were referred by...

Never change a *y* to *i* and add *es* to create the plural ending of a name.

The Peabodys (*not* Peabodies)

numbers (including years)

Add *s* without an apostrophe. Exception: With single numerals, add *'s*.

500s

She is in her 20s.

6's and 7's

abbreviated units of measure

The singular and plural forms are the same. Do not add *s* or *'s*.

> 5 mg
>
> 8 mL

irregular forms

Some words change form in the plural. Consult medical and English dictionaries for guidance.

> | *singular* | *plural* |
> |------------|----------|
> | child | children |
> | woman | women |

Some words are always singular in usage.

> ascites
>
> herpes
>
> lues

> His herpes was dormant for several years.

Some words are always plural in usage.

> adnexa
>
> genitalia

> The left adnexa were removed along with the uterus.

Some words retain the same form, whether singular or plural.

> biceps
>
> facies

series

forceps

scissors

Decubitus is an adjective, not a noun, and does not have a plural form. The plural form of *decubitus ulcer* is *decubitus ulcers*.

D: decubiti

T: decubitus ulcers

medical terms derived from Latin or Greek

General rules follow. Consult appropriate medical dictionaries for additional guidance.

words ending in -en

Change text ending to *-ina*.

foramen   foramina

words ending in -a

Add *-e*.

conjunctiva   conjunctivae

words ending in -us

Change ending to *-i*.

meniscus   menisci

embolus   emboli

Exceptions:

meatus   meatus

processus   processus

words ending in -on
Change ending to -a.

ganglion　　　　ganglia

words ending in -is
Change ending to -es.

diagnosis　　　　diagnoses

Exceptions:

arthritis　　　　arthritides
epididymis　　　　epididymides

words ending in -um
Change ending to -a.

diverticulum　　　diverticula

miscellaneous
The plural forms of Latin terms that consist of a noun-adjective combination are often difficult to determine. (In Latin, the adjective must agree in number, gender, and case with the noun it modifies.) In the following list we show such terms in their singular and plural forms; they are all in the nominative case.

singular	*plural*
processus vaginalis	processus vaginales
chorda tendinea	chordae tendineae
verruca vulgaris	verrucae vulgares
nucleus pulposus	nuclei pulposi
pars interarticularis	partes interarticulares
placenta previa	placentae previae
musculus trapezius	musculi trapezii

Sometimes the genitive case (used in Latin to show possession) is misread as a plural, causing confusion. The following terms consist, for the most part, of a noun in the nominative case plus a noun in the genitive case.

Latin term	*English translation*
abruptio placentae	rupture of the placenta
bulbus urethrae	bulb of the urethra, bulbous urethra
cervix uteri	neck of uterus, uterine cervix
chondromalacia patellae	chondromalacia of the patella
corpus uteri	body of uterus, uterine corpus
os calcis (plural: ossa calcium)	bone(s) of the heel(s)
os coxae (plural: ossa coxae)	bone(s) of the hip(s)
pars uterina placentae	the part of the placenta derived from uterine tissue
pruritus vulvae	itching of the vulva
muscularis mucosae *or* lamina muscularis mucosae	muscular (layer) of mucosa

plus, plus sign (+)

Do not use the plus sign without a numeral.

+1, +2, +3, +4

or 1+, 2+, 3+, 4+

not +, ++, +++, ++++

in laboratory and technical readings

Use the symbol unless it will not be noticeable or clear.

3+ gram-positive cocci

range

Use the word *to* (not a hyphen) to indicate a range when the plus sign is used.

Reflexes 2+/4 to 3+/4 in the right lower extremity and 4+/4 on the left.

See range

meaning more than

Write out *plus* when it means *more than.*

At 40 plus, he considered himself old.

plus/minus

Express as *plus or minus* or *plus/minus,* not +/- or ± except in tables or test results.

p.o.

See drug terminology

positive findings

Findings that are not normal. Opposite of negative or normal findings.

Transcribe all findings, whether positive or negative.

See negative findings

positive sign (+)

Do not use except in special applications, e.g., blood nomenclature.

blood type O positive *or* O+
Rh+ *or* Rh positive

See plus, plus sign

possession

There are general and specialized rules for showing possession, as well as exceptions to these rules. Some of these rules and exceptions follow. Consult appropriate topics throughout this book, as well as other grammar books, for specific applications.

nouns not ending with s

Show possession by adding 's.

> patient's
> children's
> Jane's

nouns ending with s

If only the final syllable ends in a sibilant, add 's.

> We were not able to determine the fungus's origin.

When each of the final two syllables of a singular noun ends in a sibilant (s, x, z), add an apostrophe only.

> physicians' orders
> Moses' tablets

HINT: Let pronunciation be your guide. If you would not pronounce it as *Moseses* then you would not add another *s,* just an apostrophe.

nouns as descriptive terms

Do not add an apostrophe to a noun ending in *s* when it is used as a descriptive term instead of a possessive.

> educators conference
> business leaders meeting

In proper names of this type, follow the user's practice.

Arkansas Childrens Hospital
Children's Hospital and Health Center of San Diego
Veterans Administration

eponyms
While the use of the possessive form with eponyms remains acceptable, AAMT's preference is generally to drop the possessive form.

Apgar score
Babinski sign
Down syndrome
Gram stain
Hodgkin lymphoma

Sometimes an awkward construction calls for use of the possessive form.

This patient suffers from Hodgkin's.

hyphenated compound terms
Use *'s* after the final word in hyphenated compound terms.

Her daughter-in-law's opinion was important to her.
Her sons-in-law's opinions did not interest her.

compound plurals containing a possessive
Keep the existing possessive term singular and make the second noun possessive as well.

driver's licenses' renewal dates

individual possession, two or more individuals

Show possession after each name when possession is not joint.

> Dr. Green's and Dr. White's conclusions differed.

joint possession

Show possession only after the final name when possession is common to two or more individuals.

> Doctors Smith and Brown's conclusion was...

phrase or name combinations

Show possession only after the final word in phrase or name combinations.

> Miller and Keane's reference
>
> physician-in-chief's office

possessive pronouns

Do not use an apostrophe with possessive pronouns.

> The decision was hers, not mine.
>
> its course

units of time, measurement, and money

Use *'s* or *s'*, whichever is appropriate.

> 20 weeks' gestation
>
> 30 degrees' flexion
>
> 1 dollar's worth

P

HINT: If you can replace the possessive form with the preposition *of* without changing the meaning, the apostrophe is correct.

30 degrees' flexion =
30 degrees of flexion

5 months' pregnancy =
5 months of pregnancy

but not 5 months of pregnant,
so not 5 months' pregnant

Do not confuse the possessive-adjective form with the compound-modifier form, which takes a hyphen, or with other uses, such as *3 days ago*.

> 1 month's history *but* 1-month history
>
> 2 cents' worth *but* 2-cent piece

preceding a gerund

Use the possessive form of a noun or pronoun modifying a gerund (the *-ing* form of a verb used as a noun).

> D: We are concerned by the patient taking so long to respond to treatment.
>
> T: We are concerned by the patient's taking so long to respond to treatment.

Watch for subtle but important variations in meaning created by the use (or non-use) of the possessive form preceding the *-ing* form of a verb.

> The patient was not injured, thanks to the nurse's preventing her fall. (thanks to the *action* of the nurse)
>
> The patient was not injured, thanks to the nurse preventing her fall. (emphasis placed on thanking the *nurse*, not the nurse's action)

of phrases

If possible, avoid the awkward constructions that result when an *of* phrase is combined with a possessive noun.

> D: Dr. Smith's patient's friend was referred...
>
> T: A friend of Dr. Smith's patient was referred...

However, some idiomatic expressions use the possessive form appropriately.

> a patient of Dr. Smith's

post, post-

Post is a prefix that can sometimes stand on its own as a word (meaning *after*); it can also serve as an inseparable prefix.

> The patient should follow up 1 week post discharge.
> She is 3 weeks status post breast biopsy.
> Her postoperative pain has been minimal.

In the following example, the word *post* is used as part of a hyphenated compound modifier.

> post-mastectomy scar

See status post

pound

Equal to 16 ounces (7000 grains). Equal to 454 grams (0.45 kilograms) in the metric system.

To convert to kilograms, multiply by 0.45.

Abbreviation: *lb.* (with period and without *s*).

Write out, do not use abbreviation *(lb.)* except in tables.

Express with numerals.

Do not use a comma or other punctuation between units of the same dimension.

> 12 pounds 13 ounces

P

grammar

prefixes

Do not use a hyphen to join most prefixes, including *ante-, anti-, bi-, co-, contra-, counter-, de-, extra-, infra-, inter-, intra-, micro-, mid-, non-, over-, pre-, post-, pro-, pseudo-, re-, semi-, sub-, super-, supra-, trans-, tr ultra-, un-, under-*. Common examples are noted below. Consult appropriate references for additional guidance.

antecubital	intracranial	semicircular
antithesis	microscope	sublingual
bitemporal	midline	superficial
cooperate	nontender	supramammary
contraindication	overenthusiastic	transvaginal
counterproductive	preoperative	trivalent
defibrillate	posttraumatic	ultraviolet
extraterrestrial	profile	unencumbered
infraumbilical	pseudocele	underwear
interpersonal	reimburse	

for clarification

Use a hyphen after a prefix if it would have another meaning without the hyphen.

> re-cover *(cover again)*, recover *(regain)*
> re-create *(create again)*, recreate *(play)*

Use a hyphen following a prefix to avoid an awkward combination of letters and when it will assist in reading and pronunciation.

> re-x-rayed (*but* x-rayed again *is preferred*)
> co-workers
> re-emphasize

We then re-introduced the scope.

P

as independent words

Occasionally a prefix is used as an independent word.

> Nodules were found in the left mid and lower lobes of the lung.
>
> She is post L3 laminectomy.

with self-

Use a hyphen with compounds formed with the prefix *self-*.

> self-administered

with proper nouns, capitalized words, numbers, and abbreviations

Use a hyphen to join a prefix to a proper noun, capitalized word, number, or abbreviation.

> non-CMTs
>
> non-Hodgkin-like lymphoma
>
> pre-1991 admission

with units of measure

The metric system and SI units use prefixes to denote fractional or multiple units. These prefixes are joined without hyphens.

> centimeter
>
> kilogram
>
> milligram

prepositions

A preposition relates to its object, either a noun or a pronoun.

> The patient was taken into the delivery room. (Into *is the preposition;* delivery room *is its object.*)

Pronouns following prepositions must be in the objective case: *me, us, it, you, him, her, them.*

> between you and me
> *not* between you and I

The following is a list of common prepositions.

about	down	outside
across	during	over
after	except	past
against	for	through
along	from	to
among	in	toward
around	inside	under
at	into	underneath
before	like	until
below	near	up
beneath	of	with
beside	off	within
between	on	without
by		

president-elect

Lowercase except when used as a formal title before a name (and even then, *elect* is lowercase).

Hyphenate.

> She is president-elect of her professional society.
> They were introduced to President-elect Jones.

prioritize

A back formation from *priority*, increasingly used and accepted. Transcribe if dictated.

> We prioritized the events.

privacy

See confidentiality
    security

p.r.n.

See drug terminology

problem-oriented medical record

A system for patient care documentation that numbers a patient's problems (diagnoses, conditions) and reports on them one by one, usually in "SOAP" note format.

See SOAP note

profanities

See language to avoid

professional liability insurance

Also called *errors and omissions insurance,* professional liability insurance covers most kinds of wrongful or negligent conduct an MT might exhibit in his or her profession. There continues to be a diversity of views as to whether it is prudent for medical transcriptionists to carry professional liability insurance. Some states or employers require it for businesses providing medical transcription services.

See confidentiality
    risk management

P

progress note

An interim note in a patient's medical record, made by medical staff and other authorized personnel.

See Appendix A: Sample Reports

pronouns

personal

Personal pronouns have person and number as well as subjective (S), possessive (P), and objective (O) forms.

	S	*P*	*O*
first person singular	I	mine	me
first person plural	we	ours	us
second person singular	you	yours	you
second person plural	you	yours	you
third person singular	he/she/it	his/hers/its	him/her/it
third person plural	they	theirs	them

The personal pronoun must agree in number and gender with the preceding noun or pronoun to which it refers.

> The patient was sent to the postpartum floor. She improved steadily.

Do not use an apostrophe with possessive pronouns. In particular, be careful not to confuse *its* with *it's*. *Its* (no apostrophe) is the possessive form of *it*. *It's* is the contraction form of *it is* or *it has*.

> my conclusion
> your referral
> his review of systems
> our plan
> its significance (*not* it's)

ours *not* our's
theirs *not* their's
yours *not* your's

reflexive

Reflexive pronouns are pronouns combined with *-self* or *-selves*. They refer to and emphasize the subject of the verb.

She insisted on feeding herself.

Avoid other uses of reflexive pronouns.

D: The patient will be seen by Dr. Smith in 1 week and by myself in 2 weeks.
T: The patient will be seen by Dr. Smith in 1 week and by me in 2 weeks.

relative

Relative pronouns (*that, who, whom, what, which,* and their variations *whoever, whomever, whosoever, whatever, whichever*) refer to previous nouns as they introduce subordinate clauses.

Use *who* or *whom* to introduce an **essential** clause referring to a human being or to an animal with a name.

Use *that* to introduce an **essential** clause referring to an inanimate object or to an animal without a name. Exception: When *that* as a conjunction is used elsewhere in the same sentence, use *which*, not *that*, to introduce an essential clause.

Do not use commas to set off **essential** subordinate clauses.

The patient came into the emergency room, and she was treated for tachycardia that had resisted conversion in her physician's office.
He had 2 large wounds that were bleeding profusely and several small bleeders.
She said that the dog which bit her was a miniature poodle.

Use *who* or *whom* to introduce a **nonessential** clause referring to a human being or to an animal with a name.

Use *which* to introduce a **nonessential** clause referring to an inanimate object or to an animal without a name.

Precede and follow a **nonessential** clause with a comma or closing punctuation.

> The surgery, which had been postponed 3 times, was finally performed today.
>
> The patient's parents, who had been summoned from Europe, were consulted about her past history.

See clauses

without antecedents

Text with a pronoun that does not have a preceding noun or pronoun should be edited to identify the pronoun's antecedent.

> D: She is a 40-year-old white female complaining of nausea and vomiting. *(first sentence of report)*
>
> T: The patient is a 40-year-old white female complaining of nausea and vomiting.

pronunciation

It is common for medical transcriptionists to encounter mispronunciations in dictation, in the classroom, and among themselves. Of course, terms should be spelled correctly, not as they are (mis)pronounced.

> D: adnexae
> T: adnexa

> D: aeriation
> T: aeration

D: diverticuli
T: diverticula

D: orientated
T: oriented

D: pharnyx
T: pharynx

proofreading

Proofread all reports. MTs should proofread reports while transcribing, after completing transcription, and (when there is access to the printed copy) after printing the report.

For many MTs, there is no access to the printed report because it is transmitted electronically and/or printed remotely. In this circumstance, MTs must use their on-screen proofreading skills both during and after completion of the transcript.

Spellcheckers and grammar checkers are supplements to, not replacements for, proofreading.

Some transcription departments and businesses designate specific personnel as proofreaders. This does not release MTs from the responsibility to proofread their own work.

proportions

Always use numerals in expressions of proportions.

5 parts dextrose to 1 part water

pro time

The expanded form, *prothrombin time*, is preferable, but if the short form is used it should be written as two words: *pro time*.

psychiatric diagnoses
See diagnosis

pulmonary and respiratory terms
breaths per minute, respirations per minute
Spell out. Do not abbreviate.

> Respirations: 18 breaths per minute.
> *not* Respirations: 18 bpm.

> 21 respirations per minute
> *not* 21 rpm

Use virgules only in the following form.

> Respirations: 21/min
> *but not*
> 21 respirations/min

See virgule

primary symbols
Primary symbols used in pulmonary and respiratory terminology are the first terms of an expression and are expressed as follows.

C	blood gas concentration
P *or* p	pressure or partial pressure
Q	volume of blood
V	volume of gas
D	diffusing capacity
R	gas exchange ratio

secondary symbols for gas phase
Immediately follow the primary symbol.

Express as small capitals if possible; otherwise, use regular caps.

A *or* A	alveolar
B *or* B	barometric
E *or* E	expired
I *or* I	inspired
L *or* L	lung
T *or* T	tidal

secondary symbols for blood phase
Immediately follow the secondary symbol for gas phase.

Express as lowercase letters.

b	blood
a	arterial
c	capillary
v	venous

gas abbreviations
Usually the last element of the term.

Express as small capitals or regular capitals.

Use subscripts or place the numerals on the line.

CO_2 *or* CO_2 *or* CO2
O_2 *or* O_2 *or* O2
N_2 *or* N_2 *or* N2
CO *or* CO

physiology terms

Combine the above symbols for pulmonary and respiratory physiology terms.

PCO_2	partial pressure of carbon dioxide
$PaCO_2$	partial pressure of arterial carbon dioxide
PO_2	partial pressure of oxygen
PaO_2	partial pressure of arterial oxygen
V/Q	ventilation-perfusion ratio

punctuation

Follow punctuation rules and use punctuation to enhance the clarity and accuracy of the communication.

Do not make exceptions without being able to justify doing so.

Omit punctuation not required by punctuation rules and not needed for clarity and/or accuracy.

Consult specific entries in this book and other appropriate references (e.g., grammar book) for guidance.

pus

Liquid product of inflammation. Adjective: *pus-like*.

The wound was filled with a pus-like fluid.

See language to avoid

Q

q., q.h., q.i.d., q.4 h.

See drug terminology

quality assurance

Quality assurance (QA) for medical transcription contributes to risk management. A standard has been developed by ASTM's Healthcare Informatics committee called *E2117, Standard Guide for Identification and Establishment of a Quality Assurance Program for Medical Transcription.* This standard clearly defines the roles of the medical transcriptionist, the QA reviewer, the management staff, as well as the originator of the medical report.

quantity

Use arabic numerals for quantities expressed with units of measure. Space between the quantity and the unit of measure.

> 4 mm

If a quantity begins a sentence, recast the sentence or write out both the quantity and the unit of measure.

> D: 1.5% lidocaine was administered.
> T: Lidocaine 1.5% was administered.

quart

Liquid measure equivalent to 2 pints or 32 fluidounces. Metric equivalent is approximately 950 milliliters or 0.95 liter.

To convert to liters, multiply by 0.95.

question mark (?)

direct inquiries

A question mark is used to indicate a direct inquiry. Thus, it is used at the end of an interrogative sentence (a direct question).

Was the patient seen in the emergency room prior to admission?

indirect questions

Use a period instead of a question mark at the end of indirect questions.

The patient asked if he could be discharged by Saturday.

sentences including the word question

Use a period instead of a question mark at the end of a declarative sentence that includes the word *question*.

I question the consultant's conclusions.

polite requests

Use a period instead of a question mark to end polite requests cast in the form of a question.

Would you please change my appointment to Saturday.

questions in the form of declarative statements

Place a question mark at the end of a question in the form of a declarative statement.

You mean you were serious when you said you smoke 50 cigarettes a day?

questions within declarative sentences

Place a question mark at the end of a question that is part of a declarative sentence.

> How long will the operation take? we wondered.

series of incomplete questions

Place a question mark after each in a series of incomplete questions that immediately follow and relate to a preceding complete question.

> When was the patient last seen? Friday? Saturday? Sunday?

expressions of doubt or uncertainty

Use an ending question mark to indicate doubt or uncertainty.

Sometimes, particularly with diagnoses, a question mark is placed before a statement in order to indicate uncertainty.

Placement either before or after the questionable material is acceptable, but do not place the question mark both before **and** after.

> His cholesterol levels were high normal (or minimally elevated?).

> D: Diagnosis: Angina question mark
> T: Diagnosis: Angina?
> *or* Diagnosis: ?Angina.
> *not* Diagnosis: ?Angina?

Note: There is no space after the question mark in *?Angina.*

with other punctuation

Place the question mark inside the ending quotation mark if the material being quoted is in the form of a question. Follow *she said* or similar attributions with a comma when they precede a quoted question.

> The patient asked, "Must I return for followup that soon?"

Place the question mark outside the ending quotation mark if the quoted matter is not itself a question but is placed within an interrogative sentence.

> Do you think he meant it when he said, "You'll be hearing from my attorney"?

Never combine a question mark with a comma, or with another ending punctuation mark, i.e., an exclamation point, period, or other question mark. Thus, the question mark replaces the comma that normally precedes the ending quotation mark which is followed by "he said" or similar attributions.

> "Are my symptoms serious?" she asked.

Place the question mark inside the closing parenthesis when the parenthetical matter is in the form of a question.

> She said (did I hear correctly?) that she had 5 children, all delivered at home, and this is her first hospital admission.

Place the question mark outside the closing parenthesis when the parenthetical matter occurs just prior to the end of an interrogative sentence but is not itself in the form of a question.

> Did he return as scheduled for followup (the record is unclear)?

Q

quotations, quotation marks (" ")

Use quotation marks (" "), if available, instead of ditto marks (" ").

Place quotation marks at the beginning and end of a quotation.

If an uninterrupted quotation extends beyond one paragraph, place an opening quotation mark at the beginning of each paragraph, but place an ending quotation mark only at the end of the final quoted paragraph.

capitalization

Begin a complete quotation with a capital letter if it is not grammatically joined to what precedes it.

> Path report reads, "Specimen is consistent with microadenoma."

Do not use a capital letter to begin incomplete quotations or those joined grammatically to what precedes them.

> She says that she has "bad blood."

Capitalize the first word in a direct question even if the question is not placed within quotation marks.

> She refused to answer the question, What is your name?

commas

Always place the comma following a quotation inside the closing quotation mark.

> The patient stated that "the itching is driving me crazy," and she scratched her arms throughout our meeting.

periods

Always place periods inside quotation marks.

> The consultant's report reads, "The patient is a 21-year-old male referred to me by Dr. Wilson."

question marks

The placement of the question mark in relationship to ending quotation mark depends on the meaning.

Place the question mark inside the ending quotation mark if the material being quoted is in the form of a question. Follow *she said* or similar attributions with a comma when they precede a quoted question. (Note that no period follows the quotation; never combine a question mark with a period.)

> The patient asked, "Must I return for followup if my symptoms don't reappear?"

Place the question mark outside the ending quotation mark if the quoted matter is not itself a question but is placed within an interrogative sentence.

> Do you think he meant it when he said, "You'll be hearing from my attorney about this"?

semicolons

Place the semicolon outside the quotation marks.

> The patient clearly stated "no allergies"; yet, his medical record states he is allergic to penicillin.

British style

Note that British style calls for placing periods and commas **outside** quotation marks.

R

race

See sociocultural designations

range

Use numerals. It is acceptable to use a hyphen between the limits of a range if the following five conditions are met.

1. The phrases "from...to," "from...through," "between...and" are **not** used.
2. Decimals and/or commas do not appear in the numeric values.
3. Neither value contains four or more digits.
4. Neither value is a negative.
5. Neither value is accompanied by a symbol.

When all five conditions are met, a hyphen may be used. (*To* may be used instead, even when the conditions are met.)

> Our new office hours will be 1-4 p.m. Tuesdays and Thursdays.
> Systolic blood pressures were in the 150-180 range.
> BP was 120-130 over 80-90
> 8-12 wbc *or* 8 to 12 wbc

When any one of the five above conditions is **not** met, use *to* (or other appropriate wording) in place of a hyphen.

> 3+ to 4+ edema *not* 3-4+ edema
> reflexes 2+/4 to 3+/4
> $4 to $5 million
> -25 to +48
> Weight fluctuated between 120 and 130 pounds.

> Platelet counts were 120,000 to 160,000.

Do not use a colon between the limits of a range. Colons are used to express ratios, not ranges.

> 80-125 *not* 80:125

ratio

The relationship of one quantity to another.

Express the value with numerals separated by a colon.

Do not replace the colon with a virgule, dash, hyphen, or other mark.

> Mycoplasma 1:2
> cold agglutinins 1:4
> Zolyse 1:10,000
> Xylocaine with epinephrine 1:200,000

Use *to* or a hyphen instead of a colon when the expression includes words or letters instead of values. Consult appropriate references for guidance.

R

I-to-E ratio

myeloid-erythroid ratio

FEV-FVC ratio

rbc, RBC

See blood counts

recur, recurrence, recurrent

Not *reoccur, reoccurrence, reoccurrent.*

The patient had recurring infections.

Diagnosis: Recurrent fever.

references

MTs need and use a variety of reference materials to assist them in preparing medical reports. At various points throughout this text, the reader is advised to consult appropriate references for guidance. Criteria for selecting appropriate references should include the date of publication and the qualifications of the author(s), editor(s), and publisher. Publications produced by or promoted by medical societies or associations related to a particular topic may be especially good resources.

Do not be surprised by inconsistencies within and among even the most respected of publications. The medical and English languages, as well as the practice of medicine, are in constant development—and no author, editor, or publisher is perfect.

It is important for each medical transcription department or office to identify its preferred references in order to promote consistency among its MTs and within its reports. Every effort has been made in *The AAMT Book of Style for Medical Transcription* to reflect best practices in medical report preparation, and AAMT encourages its adoption as a preferred reference. A department notebook citing preferred references and noting any departmental exceptions is also recommended.

R

AAMT publishes a list of resources used by MTs (without making specific recommendations or assessments). Contact AAMT (www.aamt.org) for further information on this resource guide.

reflexes

Graded 0 to 4.

Express as an arabic numeral followed (or preceded) by a plus sign (except *0*, which stands alone). Lowercase the word *grade*.

grade	*meaning*
0	absent
+1 *or* 1+	decreased
+2 *or* 2+	normal
+3 *or* 3+	hyperactive
+4 *or* 4+	clonus

D: grade 2 to 3 plus over 4
T: grade 2+/4 to 3+/4

Do not use plus signs without the numeral, i.e., do not use +, ++, +++, ++++.

Knee reflexes were grade 3+/4.
not ...grade +++/4.

release of information

Release of protected health information involves both legal requirements and professional responsibility. MTs should not release information except as authorized by institutional policies and procedures, and consistent with the law. The patient's rights to personal and informational privacy and confidentiality must be respected. At the same time, courts and others may have legitimate rights to health information that MTs must recognize.

R

The HIPAA privacy regulations use the term "disclosure" for what has historically been known as release of information. A separate consent from the patient may be required for each disclosure, and audit trails are required for each disclosure made. Care should be taken to assure that all disclosures are made in accordance with current laws and rules.

See confidentiality

respiratory terms

See pulmonary and respiratory terms

risk management

Healthcare institution activities that identify, evaluate, reduce, and prevent the risk of injury and loss to patients, visitors, staff, and the institution itself.

Medical transcriptionists play an important role in risk management through their commitment to quality in medical transcription and through their alertness to dictated information that indicates potential risk to the patient or the institution, including its personnel. When encountered, such information should be brought to the attention of the appropriate institutional personnel, as identified in the institution's program policies.

Cross-references below address some of the topics that relate medical transcription to risk management.

See audit trails
confidentiality
dictation problems
editing
language to avoid
professional liability insurance
quality assurance for medical transcription

R

roman numerals

See numbers

root word

The main component of a term. Other parts include prefix, suffix, and combining vowel.

The joining of a root word with its combining vowel creates the combining form.

gastrology =	
gastr	root word
o	combining vowel
logy	suffix

endometritis =	
endo	prefix
metr	root word
itis	suffix

rpm

Abbreviation meaning *revolutions per minute*. Do not use as abbreviation for *respirations per minute*.

30 respirations per minute, *not* 30 rpm

S

s̄

Symbol for *without*. Frequently used in handwritten notes. Do not use in transcribed reports; rather, express in full: *without*.

Saint, Sainte

Abbreviation: *St. (saint), Ste. (sainte).* Use abbreviation in names of saints. Use full term or abbreviation in surnames and geographic names, according to preferred or common usage.

> Sault Sainte Marie
> St. Louis, Missouri
> St. Mary's Hospital
> Susan St. James

"same"

See diagnoses

scales

See cancer classifications
classification systems
orthopedics
temperature, temperature scales

scores

See classification systems
orthopedics

seasons

Do not capitalize the names of seasons unless they are part of a formal name.

spring

summer

autumn

fall

winter

Winter Olympics

security

Security precautions must be taken to protect health information in the electronic systems on which that information is stored and by which it is transferred. The voluntary standard published by ASTM International, *E1902, Standard Guide for Management of the Confidentiality and Security of Dictation, Transcription, and Transcribed Health Records,* takes the reader through the entire dictation and transcription process and points out areas where the record must be made secure. In addition, AAMT has published a document titled *HIPAA for MTs: Considerations for the Medical Transcriptionist as Business Associate,* which contains specific advice concerning the HIPAA privacy rule as well as guidance on protecting the security of healthcare documentation.

See confidentiality

self-

See prefixes

semicolons

In general, use a semicolon to mark a separation when a comma is inadequate and a period is too final.

independent clauses

Use a semicolon to separate closely related independent clauses when they are not connected by a conjunction *(and, but, for, nor, yet, so)*. Alternatively, the independent clauses may be written as separate sentences, but keep in mind that the semicolon demonstrates a relationship or link between the independent clauses that the period does not.

> The patient had a radical mastectomy for a malignancy of the breast; the nodes were negative. *(preferred)*
>
> *or* The patient had a radical mastectomy for a malignancy of the breast. The nodes were negative. *(acceptable)*

Use a semicolon before a conjunction connecting independent clauses if one or more of the clauses contain complicating internal punctuation.

> The left inguinal region was prepped and draped in the usual fashion; and with 2% lidocaine for local anesthesia, a radiopaque #4-French catheter was introduced into the left common femoral artery, employing the Seldinger technique.

Use a semicolon to separate closely related independent clauses when the second begins with a transitional word or phrase, such as *also, besides, however, in fact, instead, moreover, namely, nevertheless, rather, similarly, therefore, then*, or *thus*. Alternatively, the independent clauses may be written as separate sentences, but again, keep in mind that the semicolon shows a link or relationship between the clauses that the period does not.

> The patient had a radical mastectomy for a malignancy of the breast; however, the nodes were negative. *(preferred)*
>
> *or* The patient had a radical mastectomy for a malignancy of the breast. However, the nodes were negative. *(acceptable)*

S

items in a series

Use a semicolon to separate items in a series if one or more items in the series include internal commas. This usage is frequently seen in lists of medications and dosages, as well as in lists of lab results.

> The patient received Cerubidine 120 mg daily 3 times on February 26, 27, and 28, 2002; he received Cytosar 200 mg IV over 12 hours for 14 doses beginning February 26; and thioguanine 80 mg in the morning and 120 mg in the evening for 14 doses, for a total dose of 200 mg a day, starting February 26.

> His lab results showed white count 5.9, hemoglobin 14.6, hematocrit 43.1; PT 11.2, PTT 31.4; and urine specific gravity 1.006, pH 6, with negative dipstick and negative microscopic exam.

quotations

Always place the semicolon outside the quotation marks.

> The patient clearly stated "no allergies"; yet, his medical record states he is allergic to penicillin.

senior

Lowercase in references to academic class and member of class. Do not abbreviate *Sr.* unless used as part of a person's name.

> She is a senior at Marian High.
> The senior class graduates Saturday.

Sr., Sr

See personal names, nicknames, and initials

senior citizen

While a patient's age may be relevant, ageist labels such as this should be avoided.

See sociocultural designations

sentences

Use sentences to separate complete thoughts. Occasionally, a report will be dictated as a single sentence or just a few sentences. Break the report up into appropriate sentences, paragraphs, and sections.

Capitalize the first letter of each sentence (including clipped sentences or sentence fragments).

> The patient was referred by Dr. Watson.
> Abdomen soft, nontender. Bowel sounds active.
> Leads aVL and aVR were...

Do not begin a sentence with a word that must never be capitalized; instead, edit lightly or recast the sentence.

> D: pH was 7.18.
> T: The pH was 7.18.

clipped

Complete sentences are the grammatically correct form, but physicians and other healthcare professionals often dictate clipped sentences, omitting subjects, verbs, or articles. The originator may prefer that these clipped sentences be transcribed as dictated rather than edited to complete sentences. Dictated clipped sentences are acceptable when they achieve directness and succinctness without loss of clarity.

> Abdomen benign. Pelvic not done. Rectal negative.

Clipped sentences are particularly prevalent and acceptable in surgical reports, laboratory data, review of systems, and physical examination, even when complete sentences are used in the remaining sections of the report.

S

When the originator's style is to dictate in clipped sentences (throughout the report or in certain sections), it is not necessary to expand dictated clipped sentences into complete sentences unless that is the originator's preference.

When an occasional clipped sentence appears within a report (or within a section of a report), it may be expanded into a complete sentence in order to make the report (or section) consistent, provided the change is not too extensive. Likewise, when an occasional complete sentence appears amidst clipped sentences, it may be clipped for consistency.

simple

A simple sentence has a subject and a predicate (each can be singular or plural) expressing a single complete thought. It may also include multiple adjectives, adverbs, phrases, and appositives.

End each sentence with the appropriate ending punctuation (period, question mark, exclamation point).

> The patient was placed on the operating table.

When there are only two subjects, do not separate them by commas. When there are more than two subjects, use commas to separate them.

> Pacemaker wires and mediastinal drainage tubes were inserted.
> The aryepiglottic folds, arytenoids, and postcricoid space were normal.

When there are only two predicates, do not separate them by commas or semicolons. When there are more than two predicates, separate them by commas or, where appropriate, semicolons.

> He continued to improve and was discharged home on the second postoperative day.
> He continued to improve, was discharged home on the second postoperative day, and will return for followup in 2 weeks.

S

compound

A compound sentence has two or more independent (but closely related) clauses, each of which could stand alone as a simple sentence. The clauses may be joined by a comma and a conjunction (e.g., *and, but*) or by a semicolon.

Separate coordinate independent clauses joined by a coordinating conjunction *(and, but, or, nor)*, by a comma, or by a semicolon if one of the clauses already contains punctuation and the semicolon will enhance clarity.

> A sector iridotomy was done, and Zolyse was instilled.

When coordinate independent clauses are very short and closely related, they may be joined without a comma or semicolon.

> The x-rays were normal and the gallbladder was well visualized.

Use semicolons to separate coordinate independent clauses that are not joined by a coordinating conjunction.

> The specimen was sent to the pathologist for examination; he found nothing suspicious for carcinoma.

Conjunctive adverbs *(consequently, however, moreover, nevertheless, otherwise, therefore, thus)* are used between independent clauses. Precede them by a semicolon (sometimes a period), and follow them by a comma.

> The patient remained febrile; nevertheless, he left the hospital against medical advice.
> The pathologist found nothing suspicious for carcinoma on gross examination; however, frozen section demonstrated fibrocystic disease.

S

complex

A complex sentence has one independent (main) clause and one or more dependent (subordinate) clauses, which together express one complete thought.

Use a comma after a subordinate clause that precedes the main clause. Exception: The comma may be omitted if the subordinate clause is very short and the absence of a comma will not confuse the reader.

> Although it was inflamed, the gallbladder was without stones.

compound-complex

A compound-complex sentence has two or more independent clauses and one or more dependent clauses.

> The posterior pack was removed, and after the wound was copiously irrigated, the procedure was terminated.

See clauses
    conjunctions
    editing

series

Use commas to separate items in a series of three or more. Using a final comma before the conjunction preceding the last term is optional unless its presence or absence changes the meaning.

> Ears, nose, and throat are normal. *(final comma optional)*
>
> No dysphagia, hoarseness, or enlargement of the thyroid gland. *(final comma required)*
>
> The results showed blood sugar 46%, creatinine and BUN normal. *(no comma after creatinine)*

units of measure

Do not repeat units of measure in a related series unless their absence will confuse the reader.

> 140, 135, and 58 mL
>
> 4 x 5-cm mass

colon

Sometimes, a colon (:) is used to introduce a series. *See* horizontal series *below*.

semicolon

Use semicolons, not commas, to separate items in a complex series or in a series in which one or more entries contain commas.

> The patient was discharged on the following regimen: Carafate 1 g 4 times a day, 30 minutes after meals and one at bedtime; bethanechol 25 mg p.o. 4 times a day; and Reglan 5 mg at bedtime on a trial basis.

horizontal series

Capitalize the first letter of each item in a horizontal series following a colon when the items are separated by periods.

> The patient's past medical history includes the following: Chronic silicosis. Status post left thoracotomy. Arteriosclerotic cardiovascular disease. Mild chronic seizure disorder.

Lowercase the first letter of each item in a horizontal series following a colon when the items are separated by commas.

> The patient's past medical history includes the following: chronic silicosis, status post left thoracotomy, arteriosclerotic cardiovascular disease, mild chronic seizure disorder.

S

parentheses

To avoid clutter and confusion, use parentheses instead of commas or dashes to set off a series that describes what precedes it and that has internal commas.

> The patient had multiple complaints (headache, nausea, vomiting, and fever) and demanded to be seen immediately.
>
> *preferred to* The patient had multiple complaints—headache, nausea, vomiting, and fever—and demanded to be seen immediately.

A colon is another alternative to the dash when this type of series ends the sentence.

> The patient had multiple complaints: headache, nausea, vomiting, and fever.
>
> *or* The patient had multiple complaints (headache, nausea, vomiting, and fever).
>
> *preferred to* The patient had multiple complaints—headache, nausea, vomiting, and fever.

unparallel series

Also known as *bastard enumeration* or *A, B, 3*.

Correct an unparallel series by eliminating the serial-comma construction or editing the faulty portion to allow for serial-comma construction.

> D: She had fever, chills, and was dyspneic.
>
> T: She had fever and chills and was dyspneic.
>
> *or* She had fever, chills, and dyspnea.

vertical series

In a vertical series, capitalize the first letter of each entry, whether or not numbered; lowercase other words (except those that are always capitalized).

End each entry with a period.

FINAL DIAGNOSES

1. Type 2 diabetes mellitus.

2. Gastroenteritis.

sex change

A patient who undergoes a sex change operation will usually have a name change as well as a gender change. The general rule is to use the name and gender existing at the time referenced. Thus, if referring to the person before the operation, use the individual's name and gender at that time. If referring to the person after the operation, use the new name and gender.

However, because it may be difficult to determine what time period is referenced and the patient and/or provider may prefer to use the person's current name and gender even for past references, it may be more appropriate and practical to transcribe as dictated.

sexist language

Avoid sexist language by using sex-neutral terms unless a particular person is being referenced.

noun

Where easily done, convert sexist nouns and adjectives to sex-neutral terms.

> chairman *becomes* chair *or* chairperson
>
> policeman *or* policewoman *becomes* police officer
>
> businessman *becomes* businessperson

pronoun

Avoid creating new terms, e.g., *shem, shim*. Instead, use *he or she, him or her, his or her(s)*. The combinations *s/he, he/she, him/her, his/her*, are acceptable but their overuse leads to clutter, so wherever possible, edit to a plural pronoun or a sex-neutral noun.

S

Rather than using plural pronouns with singular indefinite antecedents, it is preferable to find alternative language.

Everyone reported his or her findings.
preferred to Everyone reported their findings.

shall, will

The usage distinctions between *shall* and *will* are lessening except in legal documents. Transcribe as dictated.

should, would

Should expresses obligation.

He should discontinue smoking.

Would expresses usual action.

He would light up a cigarette automatically after meals.

Use *would* in conditional past tense.

If he had not smoked for so many years, it would not be so difficult for him to quit.

SI

Abbreviation for International System of Units (Système International d'Unités). SI units are the units of measure associated with International System of Units.

See International System of Units

signature block

See formats
titles

size

Lowercase *size*.

Use arabic numerals.

size 8 shoes

slang

See language to avoid

slash (/)

See virgule

smoking history

See pack-year history of smoking

so

When *so* means *so that*, introducing a clause describing purpose or outcome, it should not be preceded by a comma. It is acceptable but not required in such instances to change *so* to *so that*.

D: He wanted to improve so he could attend his daughter's wedding.
T: He wanted to improve so he could attend his daughter's wedding.
or He wanted to improve so that he could attend his daughter's wedding.

When *so* indicates *therefore*, precede *so* by a comma if it introduces a new independent clause.

It is acceptable but not required in such instances to change *so* to *and so*.

> D: His condition was improved so he could attend his daughter's wedding.
>
> T: His condition was improved, so he could attend his daughter's wedding.
>
> *or* His condition was improved, and so he could attend his daughter's wedding.

SOAP note

One format used for patient care documentation, especially in problem-oriented medical records. The acronym *SOAP* stands for

> S   subjective *(patient's descriptions)*
>
> O   objective *(clinician's observations)*
>
> A   assessment *(clinician's interpretations)*
>
> P   plan *(clinician's treatment plan)*

See Appendix A: Sample Reports

Social Security number

Nine-digit number assigned by the Social Security Administration.

Group and hyphenate as follows:

> 099-12-3456

sociocultural designations

Although sociocultural designations need not be specified unless they are pertinent to patient care—such as in descriptive remarks to assure patient identification—they should be transcribed as dictated unless the language is inappropriate.

Do not use derogatory or inflammatory terms except in direct quotations that are essential to the report. Bring inappropriate usage to the attention of those responsible for risk management.

capitalization

Capitalize the names of languages, peoples, races, religions, political parties.

> Caucasian
> Chinese
> Filipino
> Methodist
> Republican

Color designations of race and ethnicity are usually not capitalized. However, some publications capitalize *Black* to identify African Americans.

> 75-year-old black woman
> 85-year-old white man

Sexual preferences or orientations are not capitalized.

> gay
> heterosexual
> lesbian

hyphenation

It is no longer necessary (or preferred) to hyphenate designations of Americans who are identified by their ethnicity, race, or nationality of origin, either in the noun form or the adjectival form.

> elderly Asian American man

See language to avoid

solutions
See normal saline

soundalikes

Terms that sound like other terms. Be alert so that you don't confuse such terms.

> The patient was seen 1 day ago.
> *not* The patient was seeing Juan Diego.

> A re-injury was suffered when...
> *not* Every injury was suffered when...

See Appendix H: Soundalikes

species

See genus and species names

specific gravity

Express with four digits and a decimal point placed between the first and second digits.

Do not drop the final zero.

> D: specific gravity ten twenty
> T: specific gravity 1.020

speech recognition

See editing

speed

Use numerals followed by appropriate abbreviation (or extended form if abbreviated form is not known or not commonly used).

> 80 rpm *or* RPM
> 65 mph *or* MPH

spellcheck, spellchecker

Electronic spellcheckers are supplements, not replacements, for the medical transcriptionist's responsibility to proofread documents and assure that terms within them are spelled correctly. Look-alike terms will pass the scrutiny of spellcheckers as will other wrong words that are spelled accurately. The spellchecker will also miss typographical errors that create real words.

spelling

The cardinal rule of spelling in medical transcription is to use appropriate dictionaries and other references to determine the correct spelling of both medical and English terms.

Do not accept the spelling offered by the originator (or your spellchecker) unless you already know it is correct.

Some words, English and medical, have more than one acceptable spelling. Use the preferred spelling, i.e., the spelling that accompanies the meaning in the dictionary, or if both accompany the meaning, the one listed first. When alternative spellings are listed, they direct the reader to the preferred spelling for the meaning.

When there is a discrepancy between the spelling in the medical dictionary and that in the English dictionary, use the medical spelling. For example, *Dorland's Medical Dictionary* gives no alternate spelling for *distention*, but *Webster's* dictionaries give *distension* or *distention*. In medical reports, then, use *distention*.

Some idiosyncrasies will be encountered. For example, although *curet* is preferred to *curette*, the double-t form must be used in word forms derived from the root term.

curet *but* curetting, curetted, curettage, curettement

stage

Do not capitalize *stage*.

S

Roman numerals are generally used for cancer stages but sometimes they are arabic. See appropriate references for guidance.

stat

Brief form for the Latin *statim* meaning *immediately*. There is no need to capitalize it or to follow it with a period.

> We ordered a stat EKG and serial cardiac enzymes.

state, county, city, and town names
abbreviations

Do not abbreviate state names in text when they stand alone.

> She flew here from Oregon yesterday.
> *not* She flew here from Ore. yesterday.

State names may be abbreviated in text when they are accompanied by a city or town name.

Traditional state abbreviations continue to be used, but two-letter US Postal Service (USPS) abbreviations are increasingly acceptable. Use a period after traditional state abbreviations.

Use USPS state abbreviations in addresses. Do not use a period after the two-letter state abbreviations approved by the US Postal Service.

Be consistent in your choice of USPS or traditional state abbreviations.

> Washington, DC (USPS)
> Washington, D.C. (traditional)

Do not abbreviate county, city, or town names in text or in addresses.

S

New York City *not* NYC

capitalization

Always capitalize the initial letter of a state, county, city, or town name or a resident designation.

> Boston, Massachusetts
> Bostonian

Lowercase the phrase *county of* **unless** referring to a county's government.

Lowercase generic uses, including use as an adjective to refer to a level of government.

> The county of Stanislaus includes Modesto, California.
> The County of Stanislaus held a budget hearing.
> Assessment of county highways...

Lowercase the phrase *state of* **unless** referring to a state's government.

Lowercase generic uses, including use as an adjective to refer to a level of government.

> The state of California has many geographies.
> The State of California challenged the federal mandate.
> state coffers
> state highways

Lowercase the phrase *city of* **unless** referring to a city's government.

Lowercase generic uses, including use as an adjective to refer to a level of government.

S

The same guidelines apply to *town, village*, etc.

> The city of Modesto is growing steadily.
> The City of Modesto challenged the state mandate.

Capitalize *city* or similar term only if an integral part of an official name or commonly used name or nickname, or in official references. Otherwise, lowercase. The same guidelines apply to *town, village*, etc.

> New York City
> City of Commerce (official name of city)
> the Windy City
> The town budget was reviewed.

In titles, capitalize *city* or similar term only if part of a formal title placed before a name; lowercase when not part of a formal title or when the title follows the name. The same guidelines apply to *town, village*, etc.

> City Manager Dixon
> William Howard, city supervisor
> John Smith, town councilperson

commas

Follow city or town name by a comma, then state or country name unless the city or town name can stand alone.

> Modesto, CA
> Venice, Italy
> San Francisco
> Boston

Place a comma before and after the state name preceded by a city or county name, or a country name preceded by a state or city name.

The patient moved to Dallas, TX, 15 years ago.

The patient returned from a business trip to Paris, France, the week prior to admission.

In addresses, place a comma after the city name but not after the state name.

Allentown, PA 18101

Place a comma between the county name and the state name.

Worcester County, Massachusetts

ZIP codes and state abbreviations

In a mailing address, capitalize both letters of the two-letter state abbreviation.

Place a single space (no comma) between the state abbreviation and the ZIP code.

Use a hyphen or en dash between the first five and last four digits of a ZIP-plus-four code.

Beverly Hills, CA 90210
New York, NY 10022-4033

See correspondence
geographic names
Appendix J: American Cities and States

status post

Latin phrase meaning *state or condition after or following.*

Do not italicize. Do not hyphenate.

When *status post* is used, place a space between *post* and the word or phrase following it.

status post hysterectomy
Left 5th toe gangrene, status post forefoot amputation.

See post, post-

sterilely
This is the only correct spelling.

street names and numbers
named streets
When part of a formal street name, spell out such terms as *street, avenue, boulevard, road, drive* within the narrative portions of reports and letters.

Abbreviate and capitalize such terms in the address portion of a letter or on an envelope (St., Ave., Blvd., Rd., Dr.).

JOHNSON STROTHERS
2508 SUTTER ST
MODESTO CA 95353
but
Johnson Strothers lives at 2508 Sutter Street, Modesto, California.
He lives on Sutter Street.

When used alone (without a name) or following more than one name, spell out and lowercase all such terms.

She lives down the street from the hospital.
He lives at Hyde and Sutter streets.

numbered streets

Spell out and capitalize *First* through *Ninth*; use numeric ordinals for 10th and higher.

> He lives on Third Street.
> She lives on 23rd Avenue.
> *but* 1011 E. 23 Ave.

Abbreviate compass points to indicate directional ends of a street or city quadrants in a numbered address. Do not use periods. Do not precede by a comma.

> 1500 Pennsylvania NW

For decades of numbered streets, use figures and add *s*, no apostrophe.

> the 40s, the 1400s, etc.

See correspondence
  Appendix J: American Cities and States

subcu

Abbreviated form for *subcutaneous* or *subcuticular*. When "subcu" is dictated and you are unsure which term is intended, spell *subcu* or *subcut*. Do not use the abbreviation *sub q* because the *q* can be mistaken for a medication dosage.

> D&T: The wound was closed with running subcu stitches of 5-0 Prolene.

See Appendix B: Dangerous Abbreviations

S

subject-verb agreement

A verb must agree in number and person with the noun that serves as its subject. Use a singular verb with a singular subject, a plural verb with a plural subject.

> The abdomen is soft and nontender.
> The lungs are clear.

Exception: *You* always takes a plural verb.

> You are late for your appointment.

The verb must agree with its subject even when the two are not in proximity. Be especially careful when another noun intervenes.

> The *findings* on tomography *were* normal. (*The subject is* findings, *not* tomography.)
> The products of conception were examined. (*The subject is* products, *not* conception.)
> What surprised me was that the symptoms were not typical. (*The subject of the sentence is* what surprised me, *not* the symptoms, *which is the subject of the dependent clause, so the verb is singular.*)

compound subjects

Compound subjects joined by *and* always take a plural verb, except when both subjects refer to the same person or thing.

> The date and time of the accident are not certain.
> *but* Spaghetti and meatballs was our first course.

Compound subjects joined by *or* or *nor* may take a singular or plural verb, depending on the subject situated closest to the verb in the sentence.

> Neither the kidneys nor the spleen was palpated.
> *but* Neither the spleen nor the kidneys were palpated.

HINT: A phrase or clause acting as a subject requires a singular verb.

S

collective nouns

Collective nouns may be singular or plural, and they take the matching verb.

> The family is in agreement on the patient's care. *(emphasizes the family as a unit)*
>
> *or*
>
> The family are in agreement on the patient's care. *(emphasizes the individual members of the family)*

time, money, and quantity

When referring to a total amount, use a singular verb. When referring to a number of individual units, use a plural verb.

> Three weeks is a long time.
>
> Five days have passed.
>
> In all, 4 doses were given, and 20 mEq was given this morning.

pronouns

If the subject is a pronoun, be careful to determine what the pronoun is referring to.

> He is one of those patients who demand constant reassurance. (*The subject of* demand *is* who, *referring to* patients, *not* he.)

irregular nouns

Some nouns always take a singular verb.

> The ascites was tapped for the third time.
>
> The patient's lues has progressed over many years' time.

Some nouns always take a plural verb.

> The left uterine adnexa were entirely involved with tumor.
>
> The right ocular adnexa are within normal limits.

Some nouns retain the same form, whether singular or plural.

> The left biceps was weaker than the right.
> The left and right biceps were equally strong.

> A scissors was used to cut...
> An Allis forceps was used to grasp...

> Several different-sized scissors were used.
> Both forceps were required to grasp...

> A series of tests was conducted.
> Several series of tests were conducted.

units of measure
Units of measure are collective singular nouns and take singular verbs.

> After the lab report came back, 20 mEq of KCl was added.
> 3 mL was injected

subscripts
Use subscripts only if they can be placed appropriately and in reduced size, and if technological limitations do not delete them; otherwise, place the character(s) on the line or use an alternative form.

> CO_2 *or* CO2 *or* carbon dioxide

suffixes
Some suffixes are joined directly to the root word they refer to, others are joined by a hyphen, and still others remain separated by a character space. General guidelines follow. Consult appropriate medical and English dictionaries for additional guidance.

Join most suffixes directly to the root word (without a hyphen), including *-fold*, *-hood, -less, -wise*. Consult an appropriate dictionary for guidance.

> likelihood
> likewise
> nevertheless
> threefold

A hyphen may sometimes be used to avoid triple consonants or vowels.

> shell-like
> ileo-ascending colostomy

Use a hyphen to join most compound nouns with a number or single letter as a suffix; in other instances, separate them by a space. Check appropriate references for specific terms.

> 2-D
> Billroth II
> factor V

super-, supra-

Super- means *more than, above, superior, or in the upper part of* the term to which it is joined.

> supernumerary (more than the usual number)
> superolateral (in the upper part of the lateral aspect)

S

Supra- means in a position above the part of the term to which it is joined.

> supraclavicular
> supraglottic
> supraorbital
> suprapubic
> supraventricular

Although the meanings of *super-* and *supra-* sometimes overlap, the two are not generally interchangeable. Both prefixes are generally joined directly to the following term without a hyphen, but the usual exceptions apply. Check dictionaries and other appropriate references for guidance as to the correct prefix and how it is joined.

See prefixes

superscripts

Use superscripts only if they can be placed appropriately and in reduced size, and if technological limitations do not delete them; otherwise, use an alternative, on-the-line form.

> 33 m^2 *or* 33 sq m

suture sizes
USP system

The United States Pharmacopeia system sizes, among other things, steel sutures and sutures of other materials. The sizes range from 11-0 (smallest) to 7 (largest). Thus, a size 7 suture is different from and larger than a size 7-0 suture.

Use 0 or 1-0 for single-aught suture; use the "digit hyphen zero" style to express sizes 2-0 through 11-0.

Express sizes 1 through 7 with whole numbers.

Place the symbol # before the size if "number" is dictated.

> 1-0 nylon *or* 0 nylon
> 2-0 nylon *not* 00 nylon
> 4-0 Vicryl *not* 0000 Vicryl
> #7 cotton *not* 0000000 cotton

> D: 3 and 4 oh silk
> T: 3-0 and 4-0 silk

Brown and Sharp gauge (B&S gauge)
System for sizing stainless steel sutures.

Use whole arabic numerals ranging from 40 (smallest) to 20 (largest). Thus, a size 30 suture is smaller than a size 25.

syllables
Division of words based on, and guiding, accurate pronunciation. Beware of extra syllables that slip into dictation.

Transcribe words as they **should** be spelled, not necessarily as they are (mis)pronounced.

> D: aeriation
> T: aeration

S

electroencephalographic electrodes

T refers to temporal electrodes.

Use subscripted numerals if available. Otherwise, place them on the line.

T3, T4 *or* T_3, T_4	midtemporal electrodes
T5, T6 *or* T_5, T_6	posterior temporal electrodes

heart sounds

T refers to tricuspid valve.

Use subscripted numerals if available. Otherwise, place them on the line.

T1 *or* T_1	tricuspid valve component

lymphocytes

Do not hyphenate noun forms, but do hyphenate adjective forms.

T lymphocytes *but* T-lymphocyte count	
T cells *but* T-cell count	

thyroid hormones

Place numerals on the line, or use subscripts if available.

T3 *or* T_3	triiodothyronine
T4 *or* T_4	thyroxine

TNM tumor staging system

T refers to tumor size or involvement. Place the numerals on the line.

> T2 N1 M1

See cancer classifications *for more detailed discussion.*

transcribed

T as abbreviation for *transcribed* is used throughout this text to indicate the transcribed text in contrast to that dictated *(D)*.

vertebra

T refers to a thoracic (or dorsal) vertebra.

Place the numerals on the line.

> T1 through T12

See orthopedics *for complete discussion of vertebrae.*

tables, tabular matter

Tables are formatted presentations of tabular matter, separate from the narrative presentation in a report. Abbreviations not generally acceptable elsewhere may be used in such tabular matter provided they are readily recognizable.

tablespoon

Equal to three teaspoons or one-half fluidounce.

Metric equivalent is approximately 15 milliliters.

To convert to milliliters, multiply by 15.

Abbreviations: *T, tbs, tbs., tbsp, tbsp.*

> tablespoonful
> **Note plural:** tablespoonfuls

teaspoon

Equal to one-third tablespoon or one-sixth fluidounce.

Metric equivalent is approximately 5 milliliters. To convert to milliliters, multiply by 5.

Abbreviations: *t, tsp, tsp.*

> teaspoonful
> **Note plural:** teaspoonfuls

telephone numbers

In a local seven-digit number, place a hyphen between the third and fourth digits.

For phone numbers within the US, place a hyphen between the three-digit area code and the seven-digit telephone number. Alternatively, the area code may be placed in parentheses.

> 209-527-9620
> *or* (209) 527-9620

International phone numbers require a country code, city code, and phone number. Dialing from the US, the international access code (011-) is also required, although it is not always written down.

Note: The use of periods or spaces in place of hyphens has long been the practice in other countries, and there is a trend toward this practice in the United States as well.

> 011-33-1-555-0864
> 011.33.1.555.0864

T

temperature, temperature scales

Express temperature degrees with numerals except for *zero*.

zero degrees
36 degrees
36°C

Use *minus* (not the symbol) to indicate temperatures below zero.

minus 48°C

If the temperature scale name (Celsius, Fahrenheit, Kelvin) or abbreviation (C, F, K) is not dictated, it is not necessary to insert it.

38°C *or* 38 degrees Celsius *or* 38 degrees

Use the degree symbol (°) if available, immediately followed by the abbreviation for the temperature scale. If the degree symbol is not available, write out *degrees* (and the temperature scale name, if dictated).

Note: There is no space between the degree symbol and the abbreviation for the temperature scale.

98°F *or* 98 degrees Fahrenheit

Celsius

Metric-system temperature scale, designed by and named for Celsius, a Swedish astronomer. Also known as *centigrade scale*, but *Celsius* is the preferred term.

Normal human temperature on the Celsius scale is 36.7°, often rounded to 37°.

In the Celsius system, zero degrees represents the freezing point of water; 100 degrees represents the boiling point at sea level.

Abbreviation: *C* (no period).

> 37°C
> *or* 37 degrees Celsius

Fahrenheit

Temperature scale designed by and named for Fahrenheit, a German-born physicist who also invented the mercury thermometer.

Normal human temperature on the Fahrenheit scale is 98.6°.

Abbreviation: *F* (no period).

> 96.5°F
> *or* 96.5 degrees Fahrenheit

Kelvin

Temperature scale based on Celsius but not identical. Used to record extremely high and low temperatures in science. The starting point is zero, representing total absence of heat and equal to minus 273.15 degrees Celsius.

To convert to Kelvin from Celsius, add 273.15 to the Celsius temperature.

Abbreviation: *K* (no period).

Capitalize *Kelvin* in references to the temperature scale, but lowercase *kelvin* when referring to the SI temperature unit. The abbreviation is always capitalized.

degree symbol (°)

The degree symbol (°) is generally used with temperatures. However, if technological limitations prevent the use of the symbol, spell out *degrees*.

> 37°C *or* 37 degrees Celsius
> 98.6°F *or* 98.6 degrees Fahrenheit

T

tense, verb

See verbs

tera-

Prefix meaning *1 trillion units of a measure.*

To convert to basic unit, move decimal point 12 places to the right, adding zeros as necessary.

that

conjunction

May be omitted after a verb such as *said, stated, announced, argued,* provided its absence will not confuse the reader about the intended meaning.

> The patient said she was weak and dizzy.
>
> *or* The patient said that she was weak and dizzy.
>
> *but*
>
> The patient said today that she would exercise.
>
> *not* The patient said today she would exercise. (*Without* that, *the reader cannot determine if the patient said it today or she is going to exercise today.*)

introduction to essential clause

Use *that* to introduce an essential clause referring to an inanimate object or to an animal without a name.

> The patient came into the emergency room, and she was treated for tachycardia that had resisted conversion in her physician's office.
>
> She had 2 large wounds that were bleeding profusely and several small bleeders.

HINT: To decide between *that* and *which*, remember that *that* is usually not preceded by a comma and *which* usually is.

T

When *that* as a conjunction is used elsewhere in the same sentence, use *which*, not *that*, to introduce the essential clause.

> It was determined that the dog which bit the child was rabid.

See clause

that is

Latin equivalents are *i.e.* and *viz.*

See Latin abbreviations

the

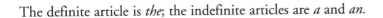

Definite article. Compare with *a, an.*

The definite article is *the*; the indefinite articles are *a* and *an.*

> *the* chair *(a specific, or definite, chair)*
> *a* chair *(may be any chair)*

See articles

thousand

Quantities dictated in the form "four point two thousand" may be transcribed as 4.2 thousand or as 4200.

t.i.d.

See drug terminology

time

abbreviations

Do not abbreviate English units of time except in virgule constructions and tables. Do not use periods with such abbreviations.

> The patient is 5 days old.
> He will return in 3 weeks for followup.
> 40 mm/h

In virgule constructions (and tables), use the following abbreviations from the SI (International System of Units). Note that no periods are used.

minute	min
hour	h
day	d
week	wk
month	mo
year	y

Abbreviate Latin expressions of time, and use periods.

> q.h.
> q.i.d.
> q.4 h.

As a side note, you will sometimes see the lowercase abbreviations *h* and *d* (without periods) for the English words *hour* and *day*. However, in medical reports, it's better to use the Latin abbreviations *h.* and *d.* for *hora* and *die*.

> q.4 h. *preferred to* q.4 h

hours and minutes

Use numerals, separated by a colon, to express hours and minutes, except for midnight and noon.

For on-the-hour expressions, it is preferable not to add the colon and 00. *See* military time *below*.

> 8:15 a.m.

> *but* 8 a.m. *or* 8 o'clock in the morning
> *not* 8:00 a.m., *not* 8:00 o'clock
> *not* 8 a.m. o'clock, *not* 8 o'clock a.m., *not* eight o'clock

> noon *not* 12 o'clock
> midnight *not* 12 o'clock

military time

Identifies the day's 24 hours by numerals 0100 through 2400, rather than 1 a.m. through noon and 1 p.m. through midnight.

Hours 0100 through 1200 are consistent with a.m. hours 1 through noon, while hours 1300 through 2400 correlate with p.m. hours 1 through midnight, respectively.

This form always takes four numerals, so insert the preceding or following zeros as necessary.

Do not separate hours from minutes with a colon. Do not use *a.m.* or *p.m.*

> 1300 hours
> 0845 hours

T

If the word *hours* is not dictated it may be added for clarity, but this is not absolutely necessary.

possessive adjectives
Use *'s* or *s'*, whichever is appropriate, with units of time used as possessive adjectives.

> 1 year's experience
> 2 months' history
> 3 days' time

time sequence
Give hours, minutes, seconds, tenths, and hundredths, in that sequence, using figures and colons as follows.

> 8:45:4.78

time span
Use hyphenated construction in a descriptive adjectival phrase expressing a time span.

> 1-month course
> 3-day period

Do not separate related time-span units by punctuation.

> Labor lasted 8 hours 15 minutes.

time zones
In extended forms, capitalize only those terms that are always capitalized, e.g., *Atlantic, Pacific.* Note: Some references capitalize *Eastern*, but some do not; be consistent.

Lowercase *standard time* and *daylight time*.

Daylight time is also known as *daylight-saving time*. Either form is correct, except that when linking the term to the name of a time zone, use *daylight time*, not *daylight-saving time*. Do not capitalize. Do not hyphenate.

> Pacific daylight time

abbreviations
Use the abbreviation only when it accompanies a clock reading.

Use all capitals in abbreviated forms, with no periods.

Do not use commas before or after the abbreviation.

> 10 a.m. EST
> Eastern standard time is...

event time
The time in the zone where an event occurs determines the date (and time) of the event.

times symbol (x)
See X, x

titles

commas
Lowercase titles that are set off from a name by commas.

> Gloria Jones, the administrative assistant, will contact the nurse.

T

compound forms
Use a hyphen in some compound titles, not in others. Check appropriate references for guidance.

> vice president
> president-elect
> editor in chief
> attorney at law

courtesy titles
Courtesy titles include *Mr., Mrs., Ms*, and *Miss*. Their use is diminishing except in letter salutations.

Abbreviate courtesy titles when they accompany a full name or surname. There is a trend toward dropping the periods following such titles.

When a woman's preference for Ms, Miss, or Mrs, is known, use it; when it is not known, use *Ms.*

> Ms White

If a woman retains her maiden name upon marriage, use *Ms* not *Mrs.*

> Susan Smith *or* Ms Susan Smith *not* Mrs. Susan Smith

If a woman takes her husband's name, use either *Ms* or *Mrs.*, whichever is her preference; if you don't know, use *Ms.*

Avoid addressing a woman by her husband's given name and surname because it is less specific for identification purposes; when such a form is used, precede it by *Mrs.* not *Ms.*

Mary Smith *or* Ms Mary Smith *or* Mrs. John Smith
not Ms John Smith

When referring to husband and wife together, use one of the following forms:

John and Mary Smith
or Mary and John Smith

Ms Mary Smith and Mr. John Smith
or Mr. John Smith and Ms Mary Smith
or Mr. and Mrs. John Smith

In salutations, use a courtesy title only with the last name, not with first and last names.

Dear Ms Smith: *not* Dear Ms Mary Smith:

When the salutation includes more than one person, precede each by a courtesy title, unless the same courtesy title applies to all, in which case its plural form may be used (use extended form, not abbreviation, for plural courtesy titles in salutations).

Dear Rev. and Mrs. Jones:
Dear Doctors Gray and White:
or Dear Dr. Gray and Dr. White:
not Dear Drs. Gray and White:

Do not use courtesy titles when other titles, degrees, or credentials are used.

Mary Jones, CMT
not
Ms Mary Jones, CMT

T

When a courtesy title for an academic degree, e.g., *Dr.*, precedes a name, do not use the degree abbreviation after the name. Use one form or the other.

> Dr. John Wilson *or* John Wilson, MD
> *not* Dr. John Wilson, MD

Do not separate a courtesy title from the name it accompanies, i.e., do not allow the courtesy title to appear at the end of one line and the name on the next line. (*For further discussion on end-of-line word division,* **see** word division.)

> After a lengthy examination of the patient, Dr. Brown concluded...
> *not* After a lengthy examination of the patient, Dr.
> Brown concluded...

false titles

A person's position of employment is not necessarily a title. Avoid making formal titles out of job position names, job description designations, occupational titles, or other labels, which always take the lowercase. **See** occupational titles *below*.

> Mary Jones, CMT, transcription supervisor

formal titles

Capitalize formal titles that precede a name and are not set off by commas. A formal title denotes a scope of authority or professional accomplishment so specific that it is an integral part of the person's identity.

> Medical Director Dr. Susan Green

Capitalize a formal title before a name even if it is a former, temporary, or about-to-be-conferred title of the individual, provided it is not set off by commas. Do not capitalize the modifying word(s) accompanying it.

former President Reagan

Abbreviate the following formal titles when used before a name.

> Dr.
> Gov.
> Lt. Gov.
> Rep.
> Sen.

Lowercase formal titles not used with a name.

> The surgeon general spoke at our meeting.

Lowercase formal titles that follow a name. Use commas to set off such titles.

> Susan Jones, director of health information services, will conduct an inservice on confidentiality on Monday.

Avoid constructions such as *surgeon Jane White*. Instead, insert *the* before the title and a comma after it.

> the surgeon, Jane White

If uncertain whether a title is formal and should be capitalized, insert *the* before it and set it off by commas.

> the attorney general, Janet Reno
> Janet Reno, the attorney general, ...

T

Lowercase titles that are not formal titles, whether they precede or follow a name. *See* occupational titles *below*.

> Ruth T. Gross, chief of pediatrics
> Ralph Emerson, St. John's Hospital administrator
> the department head, Dr. Janeway

job descriptions, job titles
See occupational titles *below*.

military titles
Capitalize when used as a formal title before a person's name.

> General Eisenhower

Lowercase such titles when they stand alone.

> The general...

The abbreviated form is acceptable only before a person's name. The abbreviation may be followed by a period, but it is not required. Be consistent.

> Gen. Bradley *or* Gen Bradley
> Capt. Kidd *or* Capt Kidd

> 1st Lt. Wilder *or* 1st Lt Wilder
> *at beginning of sentence*: First Lieutenant Wilder...

occupational titles
Always lowercase occupational titles. Do not confuse them with official titles. If not certain whether a title is occupational or official, assume it is occupational and do not capitalize it even if it precedes the name.

HINT: Only official titles can be used with a last name alone; occupational titles cannot.

T

Harry Smith, CMT, RHIA, is a medical transcription coordinator.

publication titles

Italicize or underline names of books and journals; if italics or underlining is not available, quotation marks may be used.

Place quotation marks around names of book chapters or journal articles.

Capitalize major words in titles of publications and their parts. Do not capitalize a conjunction, article, or preposition of four letters or fewer (unless it is the first or last word in the title). Capitalize two-letter verbs and both parts of dual verbs in titles.

> *Stedman's Medical Dictionary*
> "Treating AIDS in Children" is chapter 12 in this pediatrics text.
> *Wired Style*
> *The Gregg Reference Manual*

signature block titles

Use initial capitals or all caps for titles that follow a name in a signature block. Follow institutional preference.

> Ruth T. Gross, MD
> Chief of Pediatrics
>
> *or*
>
> RUTH T. GROSS, MD
> CHIEF OF PEDIATRICS

TNM staging system for malignant tumors

See cancer classifications

T

tomorrow

Be specific when referring to dates. When *tomorrow* is dictated, include the date to which it refers except in direct quotations. For example, the following was dictated on March 4, 2002.

> D: She will return tomorrow.
> T: She will return tomorrow, March 5, 2002.

ton

A US ton, also known as a short ton, equals 2000 pounds. A British ton, also known as a long ton, equals 2240 pounds. A metric ton equals 1000 kilograms (approximately 2204.62 pounds).

tonight

Be specific when referring to dates. When *tonight* is dictated, include the date to which it refers except in direct quotations. For example, the following was dictated on March 5, 2002.

> D: The patient will be admitted to the hospital tonight.
> T: The patient will be admitted to the hospital tonight, March 5, 2002.

To avoid redundancy, do not combine the word *tonight* with the abbreviation *p.m.*

> 8 tonight *or* 8 o'clock tonight *or* 8:00 tonight *or* 8 p.m.
> *not* 8 p.m. tonight

transcribed but not read

See dictated but not read

T

type

adjective

When used as an adjective, lowercase *type*.

Use arabic or roman numerals or capital letters, depending on type referred to. Check appropriate references for guidance.

> type 2 diabetes mellitus
> type II hyperlipoproteinemia
> type A personality

verb

Keyboard is replacing *type* as a verb. Avoid either term as a verb in reference to medical transcription. Use *transcribe* instead.

> The MT transcribed the report.
> *not* The MT typed the report.

type style

Regular type, also known as plain type, is preferred throughout medical transcription, with just a few exceptions when bold type or italics may be preferred or required for emphasis or to conform to a facility's model or a client's personal style.

bold type

In general, avoid bold type in medical transcription. A common exception is the use of bold type to designate a patient's allergies, although regular type is also acceptable.

> **ALLERGIES: PENICILLIN.**

Note: ASTM's *E2184, Standard Specification for Healthcare Document Formats,* calls for all major headings in the report as well as allergies (the heading **and** the substance to which the individual is allergic) to be expressed in all capital letters but with regular type (not bold).

T

italics

Use regular type, not italics, for English and medical terms as well as for foreign words and phrases that are commonly used in the English language and in medical reports.

> bruit
> cul-de-sac
> en masse
> in toto
> peau d'orange
> poudrage

Use regular type, as well, in the following instances even though italics may be called for in manuscript preparation.

> abbreviations: AFO
> arbitrary designations: patient B
> chemical elements: boron
> Latin names of genera and species: Clostridium difficile
> letters indicating shape: T-bar
> names of foreign institutions and organizations

T

under

Do not use to mean *less than*. If this meaning is intended, use *less than* instead.

> D: She weighed under 80 pounds.
> T: She weighed less than 80 pounds.

underlining

Avoid as much as possible because it reduces readability. Use regular type instead, or if type must be distinguished from regular type, use italics or boldface.

If underlining must be used, underline the full phrase, including spaces and punctuation, except the final punctuation.

United States

Abbreviation: *US* or *U.S.* Use the abbreviation only as a modifier.

> She came to the United States in 1983.
> She became a US citizen in 1989.

units of measure

metric system

System of weights and measures based upon the meter.

Metric units are increased by multiples of 10, decreased by divisors of 10.

U

Prefixes are added to denote fractional or multiple units.

deci-	one-tenth
centi-	one-hundredth
milli-	one-thousandth
micro-	one-millionth
nano-	one-billionth
pico-	one-trillionth
deka-	10 units
hecto-	100 units
kilo-	1000 units
mega-	one million units
giga-	one billion units
tera-	one trillion units

The following are abbreviations for the metric units of measure most commonly used in medical reports. Do not use periods.

cm	centimeter
dL	deciliter
g	gram
L	liter
mEq	milliequivalent
mg	milligram
mL	milliliter
mm	millimeter
mmHg	millimeter of mercury
mmol	millimole
msec, ms	millisecond

Use these abbreviations only when a numeric quantity precedes the unit of measure. Do not add an *s* to indicate plural form.

U

Do not capitalize most metric units of measure or their abbreviations. Learn the obvious exceptions, and consult appropriate references for guidance.

cm	centimeter
dB	decibel
Hz	hertz
L	liter

Use the decimal form with metric units of measure even when dictated as fractions, unless they are not easily converted.

D: four and a half millimeters
T: 4.5 mm *not* 4½ mm

D: four and a third millimeters
T: 4-1/3 mm

nonmetric units of measure

Spell out common nonmetric units of measure (*ounce, pound, inch, foot, yard, mile,* etc.) to express weight, depth, distance, height, length, and width, except in tables. Do not use an apostrophe or quotation marks to indicate *feet* or *inches*, respectively (except in tables).

4 pounds
5 ounces
14 inches
5 feet
5 feet 3 inches *not* 5' 3" *not* 5 ft. 3 in.

Do not abbreviate most nonmetric units of measure, except in tables. Use the same abbreviation for both singular and plural forms; do not add *s*.

5 in. (*use* in. *only in a table*)

U

punctuation
commas
Do not use a comma or other punctuation between units of the same dimension.

> The infant weighed 5 pounds 3 ounces.
> He is 5 feet 4 inches tall.

hyphens
Use a hyphen to join a number and a unit of measure when they are used as an adjective preceding a noun.

> 4.5-mm incision
> 5-inch wound
> 8-pound 5-ounce baby girl

numerals
Avoid separating a numeral from its accompanying unit of measure (abbreviated or not) at the end of a line. If technology allows, use a required space, coded space, or nonbreaking space between them to assure that the numerals move to the next line along with the abbreviation.

> ....5 cm
> *not* 5
> cm

series
Do not repeat units of measure in a related series unless their absence will confuse the reader.

> The daily doses were 140, 135, and 58 mL, respectively.
> 4 x 5-cm mass

U

subject-verb agreement

Units of measure are collective singular nouns and take singular verbs.

After the lab report came back, 20 mEq of KCl was added.

urinalysis

Term evolved from *urine analysis*, which is now archaic. Edit to *urinalysis*.

Use abbreviation *UA* only if dictated.

D: Urine analysis showed...

T: Urinalysis showed...

USPS guidelines

See correspondence

Appendix J: American Cities and States

U

V

verbatim transcription

Most dictation cannot be transcribed verbatim if it is to be complete, comprehensible, and consistent, since few people speak in a manner that allows conversion into printed form without at least minor editing.

Nevertheless, medical transcriptionists may be required to transcribe some or all reports verbatim. Unless the dictation is perfect (which is unlikely), the MT should retain some evidence of the directive. If the facility guidelines allow, the transcriptionist may choose to enter the statement "transcribed verbatim" at the end of the report, in order to defend the transcript in the future if necessary.

See audit trails
    dictation problems
    editing
    risk management

verbs

Verbs express action or being. Verbs have mood, person and number, tense, and voice.

mood

The indicative mood makes factual statements and is most common.

> The patient returned on schedule for a followup visit.

The imperative mood makes requests or demands.

Come here now.

The subjunctive mood expresses doubt, wishes, regrets, or conditions contrary to fact. It is the most difficult and most formal mood and usually relates to the past or present, not the future.

indicative	He is a singer.
imperative	Clean up your room.
subjunctive	If she were my patient, I would proceed with surgery.

person and number

Person expresses the entity (first, second, or third) that is acting or being. *Number* expresses whether the person is singular or plural.

first person singular	I
second person singular	you *(one only)*
third person singular	he, she, *or* it
first person plural	we
second person plural	you *(more than one)*
third person plural	they

tense

Use verb tense to communicate the appropriate time of the action or being: past, present, future, past perfect, present perfect, and future perfect. Maintain uniformity of tense, but keep in mind that tense may vary within a single report or even a single paragraph, depending on the time being referenced.

D: The abdomen is soft. There was a scar in the lower right quadrant.
T: The abdomen is soft. There is a scar in the lower right quadrant.

Tenses may appropriately vary within a single paragraph and certainly within a report.

> She was admitted from the emergency room at 8:30 p.m. She is afebrile at present. She will be given IV antibiotics, nevertheless.

historic present

Uses the present tense to relate past events in a more immediate manner. In dictation, it is common to use the historic present tense to describe patient information or treatment in the present rather than in the past. If this is done, be consistent. The historic present is not the same as the universal present *(See below)*.

> The *patient says she has* pain over the right abdomen.
> Upon examination, *there is* rebound tenderness.

universal present

Uses the present tense to state something that is universally true or that was believed to be true at the time. The universal present is not the same as the historic present *(See above)*.

> Traditional treatment modalities were used because *they are* so effective.

voice

In the active voice, the subject is the doer. In the passive voice, the subject is done unto. Most communication guidelines urge use of the active voice except when it is more important to emphasize **what** was acted on and that it **was** acted on.

V

In medical transcription, the active voice is more common in reporting observations, e.g., in history and physical exam reports, while the passive voice is more common in describing healthcare providers' actions, e.g., hospital treatment and surgery.

> The abdomen is soft, nontender.
> The patient was given intravenous aminophylline.
> The incision was made over the symphysis pubis.

Do not recast most dictation to change the voice except for those sentences that are especially awkward.

> D: The medication by him is taken irregularly.
> T: He takes the medication irregularly.

linking verbs

Verbs that link the subject of a sentence to an adjective or other complement. Most common examples are various forms of the verb *to be*. Others include *act, appear, feel, look, remain, become, get, grow, seem, smell, sound*, and *taste*.

Such verbs are followed by adjectives, not adverbs, because the subject, not the verb, is being described.

> He says the food tastes bad.
> *not* He says the food tastes badly.

split verbs

A split verb is one in which a word (usually an adverb) has been inserted between its two parts. Splitting infinitives or other forms of verbs used to be considered a grave grammatical faux pas. Traditionalists still hold to this view, but pragmatists recognize that such splits are appropriate if they enhance meaning (or at least do not obstruct it).

V

Transcribe split verbs as dictated provided they do not obstruct the meaning.

> The test was intended *to* definitively *determine...*
> He *will* routinely *return* for followup.

unnecessary verbs

In comparisons such as the following, the second verb is understood.

> The larger incision healed faster than the smaller one.

If the second verb is dictated or added, be sure to place it at the end.

> The larger incision healed faster than the smaller one did.
> *not* The larger incision healed faster than did the smaller one.

verb-subject agreement

See subject-verb agreement

Veress needle

The correct spelling is *Veress,* although many continue to use the incorrect spelling with two *r*'s and one *s.*

In the introduction dated July 1992 to *Vera Pyle's Current Medical Terminology,* the author remarks on an article written by a Dr. Veress, the developer of the Veress needle, thus confirming the spelling. (In this introduction, Pyle explains how she researches terms and arrives at conclusions regarding spelling and usage.)

versus

Abbreviation: *v* or *vs* (lowercase, no period) or *v., vs.* (lowercase, with period).

Versus is most often abbreviated when referencing a court case.

> Roe v Wade

V

vertebra

Expressed by a capital *C, T, L,* or *S* to indicate the region (cervical, thoracic, lumbar, or sacral), followed by an arabic numeral placed on the line (do not subscript or superscript). *D* for *dorsal* is sometimes substituted for *T* (thoracic).

Do not use a hyphen between the letter and the number of a specific vertebra.

Do not subscript or superscript the numerals.

> S1 *not* S-1
> T2 *or* D2

Plural: *vertebrae.*

It is preferable to repeat the letter before each item in a list of vertebrae.

> It is a lesion involving C4, C5, and C6.
> *not* ...C4, 5, and 6.
> *and not* ...C4, 5, 6.

Use a hyphen to express the space between two vertebrae (the intervertebral space). It is not necessary to repeat the same letter before the second vertebra, but it may be transcribed if dictated.

> C1-2 *or* C1-C2
> L5-S1

Veterans Administration

Veterans is used as a noun-adjective not as a possessive, so there is no apostrophe.

V

Abbreviation: *VA* (no periods).

> Veterans Administration Hospital
> VA Hospital

vice

Do not hyphenate in titles.

> vice president
> vice admiral

virgule (/)

The virgule, also known as *diagonal, slant line, slash, solidus,* is used for a variety of purposes.

alternatives

Virgules are often used to express equivalent alternatives. However, this construction can often be avoided by the use of *and* or *or*.

> a yes or no vote
> *preferred to* a yes/no vote

The *and/or* construction is particularly awkward and can be remedied in the following manner.

> We are considering surgery or chemotherapy, or both.
> *preferred to* We are considering surgery and/or chemotherapy.

See duality *below*.

V

dates

Virgules may be used to separate numerals representing the month, day, and year in tables and figures. This form may also be used for admission and discharge dates when giving patient demographic data, and for dates dictated and transcribed. As a less acceptable alterative, hyphens may be used instead of virgules.

> Admission: 4/4/02
> Discharge: 4/9/02

Note: Institutional policy, or the pre-programmed computer, may require six-digit dates for the month, day, and year (MM/DD/YY) or eight-digit dates (MM/DD/YYYY):

> DD: 04/09/02
> DT: 04/10/02
> *or* DT: 04/10/2002

In text, it is preferable to spell out dates in full, writing out the name of the month. However, if dates are used repeatedly and become cumbersome, they may be expressed as numerals separated by virgules or hyphens.

> Blood cultures were repeated on 12/3/01, 12/17/01, and 12/31/01.

When only the month and day are dictated, and the not the year, it is preferable for the medical transcriptionist to add the year, but only if it can be done with certainty and doesn't create clutter and cause confusion.

> D: The patient was seen on April 4th.
> T: The patient was seen on April 4, 2000. *(if certain of the year)*

V

duality

Use a virgule to imply duality, i.e., that the entity on each side of the virgule is the same as the other. When the two entities are not the same, use another punctuation mark, e.g., the hyphen. ***See*** and/or *above.*

> physician/patient *(one person; physician as patient)*
> physician-patient relationship *(two people)*

> employer-employee relationship
> *not* employer/employee relationship

fractions

Use a virgule to separate the numerator from the denominator in fractions.

> 4/5
> 2/3
> 1/2

over

Use a virgule to express *over* in expressions such as the following:

> blood pressure 160/100
> grade 1/4 murmur

per

To express *per* with a virgule, there must be at least one specific numeric quantity, and the element immediately on each side of the virgule must be either a specific numeric quantity or a unit of measurement.

V

Do not use a virgule when a unit of measure does not have an acceptable abbreviated form, when a prepositional phrase intervenes between the elements between *per*, or when a nontechnical phrase is used.

> Sed rate: 52 mm/h
> 120 beats per minute *not* 120 beats/min
>
> She takes 5 mg of Valium per day.
> *not* She takes 5 mg of Valium/day.
>
> She weighs in 3 days per week.
> *not* She weighs in 3 d/wk.

Avoid using more than one virgule per expression to reduce clutter and enhance readability.

> 4 mL/kg per minute *not* 4 mL/kg/min

Exception: It is very common in cancer protocols to use two virgules in an expression of a dosage.

> The patient was begun on a lymphoma protocol that included doxorubicin 25 mg/m^2/day on days 1 and 15...

visual acuity

Express with arabic numerals separated by a virgule.

> Visual acuity: 20/200 corrected to 20/40.

accent mark

See accent marks

virus names

Viruses have both vernacular (common) and official names. Do not capitalize most common or vernacular virus names, except for eponyms associated with them.

>   herpesvirus
>   herpes simplex virus
>   Epstein-Barr virus

Capitalize official (family, subfamily) names. The endings *-idae* and *-inae* indicate such terms.

>   Parvoviridae *(family)*
>   Oncovirinae *(subfamily)*

The ending *-virus* usually indicates an official term but sometimes indicates a vernacular term. The vernacular usage usually makes *virus* a separate word, but not always.

>   Rotavirus *(family)*
>   parvovirus *(vernacular)*
>   rubella virus *(vernacular)*

When two or more forms are acceptable, choose one and use it consistently.

>   papovavirus *or* PaPoVa virus

Some virus names derive from combinations of words, as a kind of acronym. Some that were originally capitalized are now preferred lowercase.

>   echovirus (**e**nteric **c**ytopathic **h**uman **o**rphan virus; *previously expressed as* ECHOvirus)

V

Use arabic numerals in most series designations of virus, but use roman numerals in the HTLV series.

> LAV-1 (lymphadenopathy-associated virus type 1)
> HTLV-II (human T-cell lymphotropic virus type II)

visual acuity

Express with arabic numerals separated by a virgule.

> His visual acuity of 20/200 is corrected to 20/40.

vitamins

See drug terminology

volume

Use a lowercase *x* and numerals in expressions of volume.

> 2 x 3 x 4 m cu
> *or* 2 x 3 x 4 m^3

Use liters to show liquid or gas volume, cubic meters to show solid volumes.

> 3 L
> 4 m cu *or* 4 m^3

vulgarities

See language to avoid

V

W

wbc, WBC

See blood counts

weight

Express with numerals.

Spell out *pounds* and *ounces* except in tables.

Do not separate the pounds expression from the ounces expression by *and*, a comma, or other punctuation when they are a unit.

> The infant weighed 4 pounds 5 ounces.
> *not* 4 lb. 5 oz., *not* 4 pounds, 5 ounces

Use abbreviations for metric units of weight.

> 5 g
> 24 kg

whether or not

Drop *or not* when *whether* means *if,* which implies an alternative. Retain *or not* when the intended meaning is *regardless.* Determine whether to retain *or not* by testing the sentence without it.

> Some use *or not* whether or not it is needed.
> We will determine whether (if) he needs surgery after the lab results are available.

W

However, this is such a fine point of good grammar that it is perfectly acceptable to transcribe *whether or not* when it is dictated.

which, that
See clauses

who, whom

Use *who* or *whom* to refer to a person as an individual, or to an animal with a name. Use *who* as the subject of a sentence or clause.

> The patient is a 67-year-old white female who injured her back after strenuous exercise.

Note: *That* is used when referring to the identity of a group.

> She is the type of person that needs to proceed with caution when exercising.

Use *whom* as the object of a verb or preposition.

> He could not say who had done what to whom.

HINT: When deciding between the subject and object, *who* does something (subject) and *whom* has something done to him or her (object).

who's, whose

> The contraction *who's* is used for *who is* or *who has*.

> Who's questioning my diagnosis?

> *Whose* is the possessive form of *who*.

> Whose idea was it to admit this patient?

W

width

Express with numerals.

    4 cm wide

will, shall

Usage distinctions between *will* and *shall* are lessening except in legal documents.

Transcribe as dictated.

word division

Avoiding end-of-line word division facilitates both communication and transcription: the reader of the document does not lose the flow of reading and meaning, and the medical transcriptionist does not have to hesitate or stop to determine correct word division.

If you choose to use end-of-line word division, follow the rules for medical and English word division.

Medical words are generally divided between word parts. It is preferable to divide after a prefix or before a suffix rather than within any word part.

For example, if *esophagogastroduodenoscopy* must be split at the end of a line, choose one of the following.

    ....esophago-
    gastroduodenoscopy
    or
    ....esophagogastro-
    duodenoscopy

W

In general, the system used in most US dictionaries is to divide words between syllables and according to pronunciation. Consult English dictionaries for guidance with specific terms.

Do not divide a word in a manner that will not leave at least three characters (including the hyphen) on the first line and at least three characters (including a punctuation mark, if any) on the next line.

incorrect:	a-cetic
correct:	acetic (no division)

Do not divide words of one syllable. Remember that when *-ed* is added to some words, they remain one syllable and so must not be divided.

crossed

Do not divide abbreviations or acronyms.

wbc's
MAST
BiPAP

Do not divide words at the end of more than two consecutive lines.

Do not divide the word at the end of the last line of a paragraph or at the end of the last line on a page.

proper names
Avoid dividing proper names. If this cannot be avoided, break between words, not within them.

W

...................................Presbyterian
Hospital
rather than...................................Presby-
terian Hospital

In particular, avoid dividing a person's name. If this cannot be avoided, make the break between the middle initial and last name or between the first and last names if there is no middle initial.

...................................John F.
Kennedy
not...................................John
F. Kennedy

Avoid separating a title from a proper name.

...................................Dr. Livingstone
not...................................Dr.
Livingstone

...................................Dr. Stanley Livingstone
not...................................Dr.
Stanley Livingstone

...................................Stanley Livingstone, MD
or...................................Stanley
Livingstone, MD
not...................................Stanley Livingstone,
MD

W

numbers

Do not divide numbers.

3400

45,587

Do not separate parts of a measurement, and do not separate a numeral from its unit of measure.

6 x 3 x 3 cm

When possible, do not separate numerals from the terms they accompany. Do not allow a numeral to end on one line and its accompanying term to begin the next.

.....................................grade 2.

not...................................grade

2.

widows and orphans

Avoid starting a new paragraph at the bottom of a page and going to a new page after only one line (called *widow* in printer's parlance). Instead, move the start of the paragraph to the next page.

By the same token, avoid having only a header and signature or only the last line of a paragraph (called *orphan*) on a new page. The solution is to bring forward one or two lines of the last paragraph from the previous page.

World War I, World War II

Capitalize the words and use roman numerals.

Abbreviations: *WWI* and *WWII*.

W

X

X, x

Use only with numerals. Use a lowercase *x* in expressions of area and volume, as a multiplication symbol, and when it takes the place of the word *times*.

A capital *X* is generally used to express magnification.

> X30 magnification

x meaning by (dimensions)

Use a lowercase *x* to express *by* in dimensions.

Space before and after the *x*.

> 13 x 2 cm

x meaning for

When the word "times" is dictated and can be translated as *for*, it should be transcribed as *for* rather than using *times* or *x*.

> D: The patient was given antibiotics to take *times* 2 weeks.
> T: The patient was given antibiotics to take *for* 2 weeks.

x meaning times

When the word "times" is dictated and means the number of times a thing was done, the letter *x* can be used.

X

To keep this expression together and easily read as a unit, do not place a space after the *x*.

> D: Blood cultures were negative times 3.
> T: Blood cultures were negative x3.

Use the symbol *x* meaning *times* only when the *x* precedes a numeral.

> D: Demerol was administered 3 times.
> T: Demerol was administered 3 times. *not* ...3x.

XML

XML (extensible markup language) is a set of guidelines for designing text formats that allows for structuring of data and better functionality in the display, manipulation, storage, and retrieval of electronic information. It makes use of tags and attributes, just as HTML does; however, XML is more flexible. It is gaining a strong reputation and widespread use in health care, both in medical transcription and in structured data entry.

x-ray

Refers both to the radiologic process and to the radiation particles.

Whether used as a noun, verb, or adjective, lowercase and hyphenate.

> His x-ray was not in the jacket. *(noun)*
> He was x-rayed yesterday. *(verb)*
> His x-ray films have been lost. *(adjective)*

Capitalize *x-ray* only when it is the first word in a sentence.

> X-ray films showed...

Avoid using the prefix *re-* with *x-ray*. Edit instead.

> x-ray again
> *preferred to* re-x-ray
> *not* rex-ray

X

Y

yard

Equal to three feet. Metric equivalent: approximately 0.91 meter.

To convert to meters, multiply by 0.91.

Do not use abbreviation *(yd.)* except in tables.

Do not use commas or other punctuation between units of the same dimension.

Express with arabic numerals.

> 3 yards 2 feet 10 inches

years, decades, centuries

years

Use numerals to express specific years. When referring to a single year without the century, precede it by an apostrophe.

> 2001
> '99

decades

Express with numerals except in special circumstances.

Add *s* (without an apostrophe) to form the numeric plural.

> The patient was well until the 1990s.

Use a preceding apostrophe in shortened numeric expressions relating to decades of the century ('90s), but omit the preceding apostrophe in expressions relating to decades of age (80s).

> He grew up in the '70s.
> He is in his 50s.

Spell out and capitalize special references for decades.

> the Roaring Twenties, the Gay Nineties

centuries
Lowercase *century*.

Spell out and lowercase century numbers *first* through *ninth*; use numerals for 10th and higher.

> third century
> 21st century

Use a hyphen when *century* is part of a compound modifier.

> 20th-century music

For proper names, use the form preferred by the organization.

> The Twenty-First Century Foundation
> 20th Century Fox

at beginning of sentence

Although numerals are generally not used to begin a sentence, it is acceptable to begin a sentence with a four-digit year expressed with numerals.

> 2001 was a catastrophic year for his health.

Note: Although it's acceptable to begin a sentence with a year, it is better to recast the sentence if possible

> The year 2001 was catastrophic for his health.

yesterday

Be specific when referring to dates. When "yesterday" is dictated, include the date to which it refers except in direct quotations. For example, the following was dictated on March 5, 2002.

> D: The patient was first seen yesterday.
> T: The patient was first seen yesterday, March 4, 2002.

your, yours

See pronouns

Z

zero
    See numerals

zip codes
    See correspondence

Appendices

Appendix A
Sample Reports

History and Physical

CHIEF COMPLAINT
Status post motor vehicle accident.

HISTORY OF PRESENT ILLNESS
The patient is a 17-year-old white male who is status post a high-speed motor vehicle accident in which he was ejected from the vehicle. He denies loss of consciousness, although the EMT people report that he did have loss of consciousness. The patient was stable en route. Upon arrival, he complained of headache.

PAST MEDICAL HISTORY
Medical: None. Surgical: None.

REVIEW OF SYSTEMS
Cardiac: No history.
Pulmonary: Some morning cough (patient is a smoker).

MEDICATIONS
None.

ALLERGIES
No known drug allergies.

(continued)

History and Physical, Page 2

PHYSICAL EXAMINATION
VITAL SIGNS: Blood pressure 120/80, pulse 82, respirations 20, temperature 36.8°.
HEENT: Contusion over right occiput. Tympanic membranes benign.
NECK: Nontender.
CHEST: Atraumatic, nontender.
LUNGS: Clear to auscultation and percussion.
ABDOMEN: Flat, soft, and nontender.
BACK: Atraumatic, nontender.
PELVIS: Stable.
EXTREMITIES: Contusion over right forearm. No underlying bone deformity or crepitus.
RECTAL: Normal sphincter tone; guaiac negative.
NEUROLOGIC: Glasgow coma scale 15. Pupils equal, round, reactive to light. Patient moves all 4 extremities without focal deficit.

DIAGNOSTIC DATA
Serial hematocrits 44.5, 42.4, and 40.4. White blood count 6.3. Ethanol: None. Amylase 66. Urinalysis normal. PT 12.6, PTT 29. Chem-7 panel within normal limits. X-rays of cervical spine and lumbosacral spine within normal limits. X-rays of pelvis and chest within normal limits.

ASSESSMENT
1. Closed head injury.
2. Rule out intra-abdominal injury.

PLAN
The patient will be admitted to the trauma surgery service for continued evaluation and treatment for closed head injury as well as possible intra-abdominal injury.

Consultation

REASON FOR CONSULTATION
This 92-year-old female states that last night she had a transient episode of slurred speech and numbness of her left cheek for a few hours. However, the chart indicates that she had recurrent TIAs 3 times yesterday, each lasting about 5 minutes, with facial drooping and some mental confusion. She had also complained of blurred vision for several days. She was brought to the emergency room last night, where she was noted to have a left carotid bruit and was felt to have recurrent TIAs. The patient is on Lanoxin, amoxicillin, Hydergine, Cardizem, Lasix, Micro-K, and a salt-free diet. She does not smoke or drink alcohol.

Admission CT scan of the head showed a densely calcified mass lesion of the sphenoid bone, probably representing the benign osteochondroma seen on previous studies. CBC was normal, aside from a hemoglobin of 11.2. ECG showed atrial fibrillation. BUN was 22, creatinine normal, CPK normal, glucose normal, electrolytes normal.

PHYSICAL EXAMINATION
On examination, the patient is noted to be alert and fully oriented. She has some impairment of recent memory. She is not dysphasic, nor is she apraxic. Speech is normal and clear. The head is noted to be normocephalic. Neck is supple. Carotid pulses are full bilaterally, with left carotid bruit. Neurologic exam shows cranial nerve function II through XII to be intact, save for some slight flattening of the left nasolabial fold. Motor examination shows no drift of the outstretched arms. There is no tremor or past-pointing. Finger-to-nose and heel-to-shin performed well bilaterally. Motor showed intact neuromuscular tone, strength, and coordination in all limbs. Reflexes 1+ and symmetrical, with bilateral plantar flexion, absent jaw jerk, no snout. Sensory exam is intact to pinprick, touch, vibration, position, temperature, and graphesthesia.

(continued)

Consultation, Page 2

IMPRESSION

Neurological examination is normal, aside from mild impairment of recent memory, slight flattening of the left nasolabial fold, and left carotid bruit. She also has atrial fibrillation, apparently chronic. In view of her age and the fact that she is in chronic atrial fibrillation, I would suspect that she most likely has had embolic phenomena as the cause of her TIAs.

RECOMMENDATIONS

I would recommend conservative management with antiplatelet agents unless a near-occlusion of the carotid arteries is demonstrated, in which case you might consider it best to do an angiography and consider endarterectomy. In view of her age, I would be reluctant to recommend Coumadin anticoagulation. I will be happy to follow the patient with you.

Operation

PREOPERATIVE DIAGNOSES
1. Right spontaneous pneumothorax secondary to barometric trauma.
2. Respiratory failure.
3. Pneumonia with sepsis.

POSTOPERATIVE DIAGNOSES
1. Right spontaneous pneumothorax secondary to barometric trauma.
2. Respiratory failure.
3. Pneumonia with sepsis.

NAME OF OPERATION
Right chest tube insertion.

INDICATIONS
Spontaneous right pneumothorax secondary to barometric trauma from increased
PEEP. An early morning chest x-ray showed approximately 30% pneumothorax
on the right.

INFORMED CONSENT
Not obtained. This patient is obtunded, intubated, and septic. This is an emergent
procedure with two-physician emergency consent signed and on the chart.

PROCEDURE
The patient's right chest was prepped and draped in sterile fashion. The site of
insertion was anesthetized with 1% Xylocaine, and an incision was made. Blunt
dissection was carried out 2 intercostal spaces above the initial incision site. The chest
wall was opened, and a 32-French chest tube was placed into the thoracic cavity after
examination with the finger, making sure that the thoracic cavity had been entered
correctly. The chest tube was placed on wall suction and subsequently sutured in
place with 0 silk. A postoperative chest x-ray is pending at this time. The patient
tolerated the procedure well and was taken to the recovery room in stable condition.

(continued)

Operation, Page 2

ESTIMATED BLOOD LOSS
10 mL.

COMPLICATIONS
None.

Discharge Summary

ADMITTING DIAGNOSES
1. Second-degree heart block with 2:1 conduction.
2. Right bundle branch block.
3. Left anterior fascicular block.
4. Adult-onset diabetes.

HISTORY OF PRESENT ILLNESS
The patient is a 69-year-old white female who has been followed in my clinic for adult-onset diabetes. She is known to have a right bundle branch block and left anterior fascicular block on previous EKG. She presented to my office complaining of increased lethargy over the preceding week.

PHYSICAL EXAMINATION
Physical exam demonstrated bradycardia with pulse in the 40s. EKG revealed second-degree heart block with 2:1 conduction and a ventricular rate in the 40s. The patient denied any light-headedness, syncope, chest pain, shortness of breath, palpitations, history of myocardial infarction, or rhythm disturbance.

HOSPITAL COURSE
The patient was admitted directly to the hospital and admitted to a monitored floor. MI was ruled out, and cardiology consult was obtained. At that time, it was felt that the patient was in need of a permanent pacemaker. She underwent dual-chamber pacemaker insertion on the following day without complications. She has done well postoperatively, without any symptoms, and has remained in normal sinus rhythm with pacer capturing throughout observation. She is presently without complaints except for some nasal congestion and tenderness over the pacer insertion site. However, there is no erythema or discharge at the operative site. The patient is clinically stable for discharge.

(continued)

Discharge Summary, Page 2

DISCHARGE MEDICATIONS
1. Ecotrin 1 p.o. b.i.d. with meals.
2. Keflex 500 mg p.o. q.i.d. for 4 days.
3. Iron sulfate 325 mg p.o. b.i.d.

PLAN
The patient is to see me again in 2 weeks. She will call if symptoms recur.

Progress Note

The patient is being seen today in followup for a bad cough, sinus congestion, and nasal discharge, worse since his last visit. He also complains of a sore on the bottom of his right foot, and he has a bulge in the left groin.

PHYSICAL EXAM
HEENT shows posterior pharyngeal drainage. The neck is supple, with tender adenopathy. TMs are clear. Lungs have some forced expiratory rhonchi. Examination of the bottom of the right foot shows a corn; I pared away some of the overlying callus. Valsalva maneuver shows a prominent left inguinal hernia; testicular exam is normal.

IMPRESSION
1. Sinusitis.
2. Corn, right foot.
3. Left inguinal hernia.

PLAN
We put him on amoxicillin 250 mg t.i.d. for 10 days. Advised him to pare the corn and use a Dr. Scholl's foot pad. We will refer him to a general surgeon regarding the left inguinal hernia. Return in 2 weeks if sinusitis is not improved.

NOTE: *In order to conserve space in the chart, some physician offices, clinics, and other healthcare facilities format their progress notes by using section headings followed by colons, with findings beginning on the same line.*

SOAP Note

SUBJECTIVE
Jennifer is brought in for a 6-month checkup. She is doing very well. She is seeing Dr. Green for evaluation of her feet. He gave her a clean bill of health. She is on breast milk as well as cereal.

OBJECTIVE
HEENT exam is normal. Lungs are clear. Cardiac examination is within normal limits. Musculoskeletal exam is normal. Abdomen is benign. Genitalia are normal.

ASSESSMENT
Normal exam.

PLAN
Continue breast-feeding; no dietary modifications are necessary. DPT and HIB will be given.

NOTE: *In order to conserve space in the chart, some physician offices, clinics, and other healthcare facilities format their SOAP notes by using section headings followed by colons, with findings beginning on the same line.*

EEG

DESCRIPTION
This is the record in a 12-month-old infant on no regular medications, who received chloral hydrate before the test. The EEG is well organized and shows symmetrical activity of normal amplitude, which is persistent throughout. There is no focal or paroxysmal abnormality. Provocative procedures were not carried out. The child remained asleep throughout most of the recording.

IMPRESSION
Normal electroencephalogram.

Radiology

THYROID UPTAKE AND SCAN
Uptake is markedly elevated at 82% at 24 hours. Images show that the left lobe is considerably enlarged, about 5 times normal size, whereas the right lobe is about normal in size. There is uniform uptake throughout both lobes.

IMPRESSION
The findings are consistent with Graves disease, with asymmetric involvement of the lobes, the left being quite enlarged, whereas the right is not enlarged.

Flow Cytometry

Examination of Wright-stained cytoprep slides of the submitted bone marrow specimen shows a predominant population of maturing myeloid cells with smaller numbers of maturing erythroid cells. Only rare small lymphocytes are observed. No prominent abnormal lymphocytic population is identified.

By flow cytometric immunophenotyping, within the lymphocytic region, there is a preponderance of T lymphocytes with only a small number of B lymphocytes. No monoclonal IgM-lambda-expressing B-lymphocytic population is identified by this flow cytometric study. Nevertheless, these findings should be correlated with the bone marrow biopsy for definitive diagnosis (since some aggregates of lymphoma, especially paratrabecular lymphoma, may not be very well aspirated).

Cytology

SPECIMEN
Vaginal smear.

CLINICAL DATA
Postmenopausal vaginal bleeding.

GROSS DESCRIPTION
Received is 1 alcohol-fixed smear.

MICROSCOPIC DESCRIPTION
One Papanicolaou-stained smear is examined. The smear is highly cellular, consisting predominantly of superficial vaginal/exocervical epithelial cells intermixed with large numbers of neutrophils. Occasional trichomonas organisms are seen. No dysplastic cells are seen.

DIAGNOSIS
Pap smear showing marked acute inflammation with Trichomonas vaginalis being present (Pap smear, vagina).

Pathology

SPECIMEN
Fine-needle aspiration, right kidney.

CLINICAL DATA
Hypertension workup, asymptomatic right renal mass.

GROSS DESCRIPTION
In the department of radiology, under CT guidance, Dr. Blank performed a single pass into a right kidney mass. This resulted in production of less than 1 mL of bloody fluid. From this fluid were created 3 air-dried smears and 4 alcohol-fixed smears. In addition, the syringe and needle were rinsed in B-5 solution for producing a bloody slur totaling approximately 0.75 mL. This material will be filtered through a tea bag and submitted in its entirety in a single cassette.

MICROSCOPIC DESCRIPTION
Four Papanicolaou-stained smears, 3 Wright-stained smears, and 3 H&E-stained sections from a B-5 fixed cell button are reviewed. Seen are rather large clusters of cohesive, moderate-sized cells which are oval to spindle shaped. These cells contain nongranular, nonvacuolated cytoplasm, and cytoplasmic borders are indistinct. Gland-like lumina and evidence of squamous differentiation are lacking, and no significant areas of necrosis are found. The nuclei are rounded to oval and show a finely granular pattern of chromatin staining. Other nuclei show prominent euchromatin. Nuclei containing prominent nucleoli are not found. There is minimal nuclear pleomorphism noted, and virtually no mitotic figures are encountered. No papillary structures are seen. No calcifications are encountered. Metaplastic bone and cartilage formation are not found. No pigmentation is noted.

DIAGNOSIS
Renal cell carcinoma (hypernephroma), right kidney.

Autopsy

Patient was a 70-year-old white male with a history of adenocarcinoma of the right upper lobe, treated with lobectomy in 1985, and coronary artery disease, treated with coronary artery bypass graft in 1986. The patient presented to University Medical Center in October of 1988 with mental status changes and was found to have a right frontal lobe metastasis. The patient received steroids and x-ray therapy at that time and was discharged to home. He returned to our medical center on the 19th of October with decreasing mental status and shortness of breath. The patient was found to have a left upper lobe pneumonia and possible right lower lobe pneumonia, urinary tract infection, sinus tachycardia, ventricular ectopy, and mental status changes. He was admitted for antibiotic therapy and supportive care. The patient was made DNR (do not resuscitate) and developed agonal rhythm early on the morning of 21 October and quietly expired.

GROSS AUTOPSY FINDINGS
The body is that of a cachectic white male appearing the stated age of 70 years, measuring approximately 5 feet 8 inches in height and weighing approximately 130 pounds. Hair is white with bitemporal baldness. The eyes are of a brownish-gray color, with 3-mm pupils. The nose is unremarkable. The mouth is opened and edentulous. The neck shows the trachea to be in the midline. There is no palpable cervical adenopathy. The thorax is symmetrical. There is a well-healed midline chest incision measuring 29 cm in length and a well-healed incision at the right fourth intercostal space measuring 21 cm. The abdomen is flat. There are right and left well-healed inguinal incisions measuring 12 cm each. There is no evidence of ascites, organomegaly, or palpable masses. The extremities reveal petechiae and scabs over both arms, abrasions over both knees, and petechiae over both ankles. There are puncture wounds noted at the right and left wrists and antecubital fossae and over the right ankle. The genitalia are those of a normal adult circumcised male. The back discloses a moderate amount of livor mortis, and a mid-thoracic spine and sacral decubitus. Rigor mortis is present in the upper and lower extremities.

(continued)

Autopsy, Page 2

INTERNAL EXAMINATION

The usual Y-shaped incision is made, disclosing musculature of normal hydration, as well as a panniculus measuring 0.5 cm. There is a wire suture in the central portion of the sternum. The organs of the thoracic and abdominal cavities are in their normal anatomic positions.

Thyroid: The thyroid shows a red-brown color and smooth contour. There is no evidence of tumor.

Respiratory system: There are diffuse obliterative adhesions of the pleura on the right and focal adhesions of the pleura on the left. A hydrothorax is present bilaterally, measuring less than 50 mL. The lungs weigh 1200 gm on the left and 600 gm on the right. The right lung shows a ragged, spongy consistency, with an area of consolidation in the lower lobe. The left lung shows firm, rubbery consolidation, with parenchymal cavitation in the upper lobe and a red, spongy, congested appearance in the lower lobe. Bronchi and bronchioles are lined by a thin, red-gray mucosa covered by pink, frothy material. No tumor is noted in the lungs. There is no evidence of pulmonary emboli.

Cardiovascular system: The heart weighs 600 gm and shows evidence of biventricular dilatation. The pericardial sac is densely adherent to the epicardium and shows a 2-cm abscess cavity at the AV (atrioventricular) junction, along the left lateral/posterior wall. The myocardium is red-brown and mottled and shows multifocal fibrosis in the left ventricle and septum. In the left ventricle, the myocardium measures 1.5 cm in thickness and in the right ventricle 0.5 cm, exclusive of papillary muscles. The endocardium is smooth and moist and discloses no fibrosis or petechiae. The valve leaflets are thin and pliable and demonstrate no vegetations. The circumferences of the valves are tricuspid 11, pulmonary 8, mitral 11, aortic 6. The chordae tendineae are thin, discrete, and of normal length. The left coronary ostium is patent; the right coronary ostium appears to be attenuated. The aorta and main systemic vessels show slight arteriosclerotic change with plaques.

(continued)

Autopsy, Page 3

Spleen: The spleen weighs 200 gm. The capsule is smooth. The cut surface is deep red in color and markedly hyperemic.

Liver: The liver weighs 1750 gm and is of a red-brown color. The capsule is smooth, and the organ is firm. The parenchyma is homogeneous and of a red-brown color. The architecture is intact.

Gallbladder: The gallbladder is present, thin walled, and nondilated. It contains no stones.

Pancreas: The pancreas weighs 75 gm. It is a light pinkish-tan organ that is lobular and cuts with normal resistance.

Gastrointestinal tract: There are no adhesions noted in the abdominal cavity. There is minimal free fluid in the peritoneal cavity; this measures less than 30 mL. The esophagus is patent and normal throughout; it enters the stomach in a normal fashion. The stomach is contracted and contains 20 mL of blood. There is a mesenteric tumor nodule noted adjacent to the jejunum. The appendix is present and unremarkable. The adrenals are normal in size, shape, and anatomic position.

Genitourinary system: The right kidney weighs 225 gm, and the left kidney weighs 225 gm. The capsules strip with ease. The subcapsular surfaces are finely granular and bear a few pitted scars. The right kidney shows multiple areas of yellow-tan, minute nodules measuring approximately 1 mm apiece. The renal arteries are unremarkable. The ureters are thin walled and nondilated. The urinary bladder is contracted and thick walled, containing less than 5 mL of cloudy urine. The prostate is unremarkable.

Central nervous system: The scalp is reflected in the usual manner, and the bony calvarium appears intact. The pachymeninges are thin, fibrous, and glistening. There is no evidence of previous laceration, contusion, or healed fracture. The cerebral hemispheres are rounded and reveal slightly atrophic convolutions and sulci. The venous tributaries are markedly congested. The brain weighs 1250 gm. The vessels at the base of the brain are unremarkable. The pituitary is present in its usual anatomic position. Further examination of the brain parenchyma must follow thorough fixation.

Correspondence: Full Block Format

ABC GENERAL HOSPITAL
123 First Street
Hometown, USA

August 1, 2001

Joseph Smith, MD
100 Sycamore Avenue
Modesto, CA 95354

RE: Jane Doe

Dear Joe:

I saw Jane Doe in the office today for consultation regarding her severe weakness on the left side. This has become gradually worse over the last two months. There is a family history of multiple sclerosis in a cousin and her brother. I am not convinced that is her diagnosis; however, I have scheduled multiple laboratory studies and a brain MRI.

I will be back in touch with you next week to let you know the results of this workup.

Thank you for this interesting referral.

Sincerely,

Fred Ford, MD

FF/BH

cc Mrs. Jane Doe

	Date Line
	Address
	Reference Line
	Salutation
	Body of Letter
	Complimentary Close
	Typed Signature Line
	Reference Initials
	Courtesy Copy

Correspondence: Modified Block Format Without Indented Paragraphs

ABC GENERAL HOSPITAL
123 First Street
Hometown, USA

Date Line   August 1, 2001

Address   Joseph Smith, MD
                         100 Sycamore Avenue
                         Modesto, CA 95354

Reference Line   RE: Jane Doe

Salutation   Dear Joe:

Body of Letter   I saw Jane Doe in the office today for consultation regarding her severe weakness on the left side. This has become gradually worse over the last two months. There is a family history of multiple sclerosis in a cousin and her brother. I am not convinced that is her diagnosis; however, I have scheduled multiple laboratory studies and a brain MRI.

                         I will be back in touch with you next week to let you know the results of this workup.

                         Thank you for this interesting referral.

Complimentary Close   Sincerely,

Typed Signature Line   Fred Ford, MD

Reference Initials   FF/BH

Courtesy Copy   cc Mrs. Jane Doe

Correspondence: Modified Block Format with Indented Paragraphs

ABC GENERAL HOSPITAL
123 First Street
Hometown, USA

August 1, 2001 — **Date Line**

Joseph Smith, MD — **Address**
100 Sycamore Avenue
Modesto, CA 95354

RE: Jane Doe — **Reference Line**

Dear Joe: — **Salutation**

    I saw Jane Doe in the office today for consultation regarding her severe weakness — **Body of Letter**
on the left side. This has become gradually worse over the last two months. There is a
family history of multiple sclerosis in a cousin and her brother. I am not convinced that is
her diagnosis; however, I have scheduled multiple laboratory studies and a brain MRI.

    I will be back in touch with you next week to let you know the results of this workup.

    Thank you for this interesting referral.

Sincerely, — **Complimentary Close**

Fred Ford, MD — **Typed Signature Line**

FF/BH — **Reference Initials**

cc Mrs. Jane Doe — **Courtesy Copy**

Correspondence: Memo

MEMO

DATE: August 12, 2001

TO: All Medical Transcriptionists

FROM: Martha Washington, Department of Human Resources

SUBJECT: CMT Status Verification

Due to the recent policy change that provides all certified medical transcriptionists an incentive bonus, it is necessary to verify the status of each CMT on staff.

Please provide me with your CMT number and the expiration date (displayed on your wallet-sized card provided by the Medical Transcription Certification Commission), no later than January 4, in order to adjust your payroll to include this new bonus.

Appendix B
Dangerous Abbreviations and Dose Designations*

The Institute for Safe Medication Practices (ISMP) is a nonprofit organization that partners with healthcare practitioners toward improvements in drug distribution, naming, packaging, labeling, and delivery system design. As a result of years of data collection on medication errors, working in collaboration with the United States Pharmacopeia, ISMP has developed this list of abbreviations and dose designations that are dangerous to patient safety. (Please see further discussion on this topic in the sections on *abbreviations, acronyms, brief forms* and *drug terminology*.) It is not feasible to ask healthcare workers to develop two different systems of writing—one for handwriting and another for machine printing. Therefore, although some of the problems identified here occur only with handwriting, the practices presented here should be promoted as the preferred expression.

Abbreviation/ Dose Expression	Intended Meaning	Misinterpretation	Correction
Apothecary symbols	dram minim	Misunderstood or misread (symbol for dram misread for "3" and minim misread as "mL").	Use the metric system.
AU	aurio uterque (each ear)	Mistaken for OU (oculo uterque—each eye).	Don't use this abbreviation.
D/C	discharge discontinue	Premature discontinuation of medications when D/C (intended to mean "discharge") has been misinterpreted as "discontinued" when followed by a list of drugs.	Use "discharge" and "discontinue."
Drug names			
ARA°A	vidarabine	cytarabine ARA°C	Use the complete spelling for drug names.
AZT	zidovudine (RETROVIR)	azathioprine	Use the complete spelling for drug names.
CPZ	COMPAZINE (prochlorperazine)	chlorpromazine	Use the complete spelling for drug names.

©2001 Institute for Safe Medication Practices, Huntingdon Valley, PA (www.ismp.org/MSAarticles/specialissuetable.html). Reprinted here with permission.

Abbreviation/ Dose Expression	Intended Meaning	Misinterpretation	Correction
DPT	DEMEROL- PHENERGAN- THORAZINE	diphtheria-pertussis-tetanus (vaccine)	Use the complete spelling for drug names.
HCl	hydrochloric acid	potassium chloride (The "H" is misinterpreted as "K.")	Use the complete spelling for drug names.
HCT	hydrocortisone	hydrochlorothiazide	Use the complete spelling for drug names.
HCTZ	hydrochlorothiazide	hydrocortisone (seen as HCT250 mg)	Use the complete spelling for drug names.
MgSO4	magnesium sulfate	morphine sulfate	Use the complete spelling for drug names.
MSO4	morphine sulfate	magnesium sulfate	Use the complete spelling for drug names.
MTX	methotrexate	mitoxantrone	Use the complete spelling for drug names.
TAC	triamcinolone	tetracaine, ADRENALIN, cocaine	Use the complete spelling for drug names.
ZnSO4	zinc sulfate	morphine sulfate	Use the complete spelling for drug names.
Stemmed names			
"Nitro" drip	nitroglycerin infusion	sodium nitroprusside infusion	Use the complete spelling for drug names.
"Norflox"	norfloxacin	NORFLEX	Use the complete spelling for drug names.
μg	microgram	Mistaken for "mg" when handwritten.	Use "mcg."
o.d. or OD	once daily	Misinterpreted as "right eye" (OD—oculus dexter) and administration of oral medications in the eye.	Use "daily."
TIW or tiw	three times a week	Mistaken as "three times a day."	Don't use this abbreviation.

Abbreviation/ Dose Expression	Intended Meaning	Misinterpretation	Correction
per os	orally	The "os" can be mistaken for "left eye."	Use "PO," "by mouth," or "orally."
q.d. or QD	every day	Mistaken as q.i.d., especially if the period after the "q" or the tail of the "q" is misunderstood as an "i."	Use "daily" or "every day."
qn	nightly or at bedtime	Misinterpreted as "qh" (every hour).	Use "nightly."
qhs	nightly at bedtime	Misread as every hour.	Use "nightly."
q6PM, etc.	every evening at 6 PM	Misread as every six hours.	Use 6 PM "nightly."
q.o.d. or QOD	every other day	Misinterpreted as "q.d." (daily) or "q.i.d." (four times daily) if the "o" is poorly written.	Use "every other day."
sub q	subcutaneous	The "q" has been mistaken for "every" (e.g., one heparin dose ordered "sub q 2 hours before surgery" misunderstood as every 2 hours before surgery).	Use "subcut." or write "subcutaneous."
SC	subcutaneous	Mistaken for SL (sublingual).	Use "subcut." or write "subcutaneous."
U or u	unit	Read as a zero (0) or a four (4), causing a 10-fold overdose or greater (4U seen as "40" or 4u seen as 44").	"Unit" has no acceptable abbreviation. Use "unit."
IU	international unit	Misread as IV (intravenous).	Use "units."
cc	cubic centimeters	Misread as "U" (units).	Use "mL."
x3d	for three days	Mistaken for "three doses."	Use "for three days."
BT	bedtime	Mistaken as "BID" (twice daily).	Use "hs."

Appendix B

Abbreviation/ Dose Expression	Intended Meaning	Misinterpretation	Correction
ss	sliding scale (insulin) or 1⁄2 (apothecary)	Mistaken for "55."	Spell out "sliding scale." Use "one-half" or use "1⁄2."
> and <	greater than and less than	Mistakenly used opposite of intended.	Use "greater than" or "less than."
/ (slash mark)	separates two doses or indicates "per"	Misunderstood as the number 1 ("25 unit/10 units" read as "110" units.	Do not use a slash mark to separate doses. Use "per."
Name letters and dose numbers run together (e.g., Inderal40 mg)	Inderal 40 mg	Misread as Inderal 140 mg.	Always use space between drug name, dose and unit of measure.
Zero after decimal point (1.0)	1 mg	Misread as 10 mg if the decimal point is not seen.	Do not use terminal zeros for doses expressed in whole numbers.
No zero before decimal dose (.5 mg)	0.5 mg	Misread as 5 mg.	Always use zero before a decimal when the dose is less than a whole unit.

The American Association for Medical Transcription

Appendix C
Medical Transcriptionist Job Descriptions

Professional Levels

In an independent benchmarking study of the medical transcription profession conducted in 1999 by the Hay Management Consultants (HayGroup), three distinct professional levels for medical transcriptionists were identified and described as presented below. The HayGroup is a worldwide human resources consulting firm with extensive expertise in work analysis and job measurement.

Compensation

Subsequent to this benchmark study of the job content levels of MTs, the HayGroup conducted a compensation survey, analyzing pay as it relates to these levels. (Hay's survey methodology complied with federal antitrust regulations regarding healthcare compensation surveys.) The results include information on transcription pay at the corporate level (healthcare organizations and MT businesses) and compensation for independent contractors. The data are further presented by geographic region, size of business, types of pay programs (pay for time worked and pay for production), and reward programs (benefits, etc.). The Hay report, *Compensation for Medical Transcriptionists,* is contained in a 30-page booklet, which is available for purchase from AAMT.

Appendix C

Professional Level 1	Professional Level 2	Professional Level 3
Position Summary		
Medical language specialist who transcribes dictation by physicians and other healthcare providers in order to document patient care. The incumbent will likely need assistance to interpret dictation that is unclear or inconsistent, or make use of professional reference materials.	Medical language specialist who transcribes and interprets dictation by physicians and other healthcare providers in order to document patient care. The position is also routinely involved in research of questions and in the education of others involved with patient care documentation.	Medical language specialist whose expert depth and breadth of professional experience enables him or her to serve as a medical language resource to originators, coworkers, other healthcare providers, and/or students on a regular basis.
Nature of Work		
An incumbent in this position is given assignments that are matched to his or her developing skill level, with the intention of increasing the depth and/or breadth of exposure. OR The nature of the work performed (type of report or correspondence, medical specialty, originator) is repetitive or patterned, not requiring extensive depth and/or breadth of experience.	An incumbent in this position is given assignments that require a seasoned depth of knowledge in a medical specialty (or specialties). OR The incumbent is regularly given assignments that vary in report or correspondence type, originator, and specialty. Incumbents at this level are able to resolve non-routine problems independently, or to assist in resolving complex or highly unusual problems.	An incumbent in this position routinely researches and resolves complex questions related to health information or related documentation. AND/OR Is involved in the formal teaching of those entering the profession or continuing their education in the profession. AND/OR Regularly uses extensive experience to interpret dictation that others are unable to clarify. Actual transcription of dictation is performed only occasionally, as efforts are usually focused in other categories of work.

Professional Level 1

Professional Level 2

Professional Level 3

Knowledge, Skills & Abilities

Professional Level 1

1. Basic knowledge of medical terminology, anatomy and physiology, disease processes, signs and symptoms, medications, and laboratory values. Knowledge of specialty (or specialties) as appropriate.
2. Knowledge of medical transcription guidelines and practices.
3. Proven skills in English usage, grammar, punctuation, style, and editing.
4. Ability to use designated professional reference materials.
5. Ability to operate word processing equipment, dictation and transcription equipment, and other equipment as specified.
6. Ability to work under pressure with time constraints.
7. Ability to concentrate.
8. Excellent listening skills.
9. Excellent eye, hand, and auditory coordination.
10. Ability to understand and apply relevant legal concepts (e.g., confidentiality).

Professional Level 2

1. Seasoned knowledge of medical terminology, anatomy and physiology, disease processes, signs and symptoms, medications, and laboratory values. In-depth or broad knowledge of a specialty (or specialties) as appropriate.
2. Knowledge of medical transcription guidelines and practices.
3. Excellent skills in English usage, grammar, punctuation, and style.
4. Ability to use an extensive array of professional reference materials.
5. Ability to operate word processing equipment, dictation and transcription equipment, and other equipment as specified, and to troubleshoot as necessary.
6. Ability to work independently with minimal or no supervision.
7. Ability to work under pressure with time constraints.
8. Ability to concentrate.
9. Excellent listening skills.
10. Excellent eye, hand, and auditory coordination.
11. Proven business skills (scheduling work, purchasing, client relations, billing).
12. Ability to understand and apply relevant legal concepts (e.g., confidentiality).
13. Certified medical transcriptionist (CMT) status preferred.

Professional Level 3

1. Recognized as possessing expert knowledge of medical terminology, anatomy and physiology, disease processes, signs and symptoms, medications, and laboratory values related to a specialty or specialties.
2. In-depth knowledge of medical transcription guidelines and practices.
3. Excellent skills in English usage, grammar, punctuation, and style.
4. Ability to use a vast array of professional reference materials, often in innovative ways.
5. Ability to educate others (one-on-one or group).
6. Excellent written and oral communication skills.
7. Ability to operate word processing equipment, dictation and transcription equipment, and other equipment as specified, and to troubleshoot as necessary.
8. Proven business skills (scheduling work, purchasing, client relations, billing).
9. Ability to understand and apply relevant legal concepts (e.g., confidentiality).
10. Certified medical transcriptionist (CMT) status preferred.

Appendix D
Productivity Considerations: How Much Wood Should a Woodchuck, or a Medical Transcriptionist, Chuck?

by Pat Forbis, CMT

"How much work should an average medical transcriptionist (MT) produce in a day" is one of the most frequently asked questions by managers, supervisors and others who play numbers games. To answer the question we must agree on the definition of the average MT. In my opinion, defining the average MT is like searching for the Holy Grail. If you are looking for one, good luck. In my 30 years in this industry, I have yet to meet one...one who would admit it, at least.

In 1992 I authored a popular AAMT Track column titled "How Much Wood Should a Woodchuck Chuck...and Why?" It described how variables of the day affected the outcome of work produced by the woodchuck and the MT.

With seven years of changes in the environment, the move toward an electronic patient record, and with health care itself moving forward at an almost dizzying pace, there are some things that haven't changed and aren't likely to. One of those things is a national productivity standard for MTs.

Woodchucks and MTs still have a lot of work to do, although it appears that MTs may be outpacing their furry friends when it comes to current-day demands. Both remain focused and work diligently for long periods of time, continuing to make extraordinary progress in relatively short periods of time. Given just the right amount of uninterrupted time, knowledge, and experience, both still deliver an impressive final product.

The answer to the question of how much work an average MT should be able to produce has not changed. Today, as in 1992, there is no such thing as a national average productivity level for medical transcription, and there probably never will be. You can add to that statement that there is no such thing as an average MT.

d

Consider the variables that MTs encounter every day:

Dictation

- Dictator characteristics (English as a first or second language, voice inflection, articulation skills, new or experienced dictator)
- Dictation equipment (analog, digital, controls, maintenance, media quality, rerecord or original)
- Dictation software (speech recognition technology)
- Type of report (operative, discharge, progress notes, H&P, radiology, pathology, specialty)
- Completeness of dictation (provision of patient demographics, use of abbreviations, incomplete reports or sentences)
- Difficulty factors of reports (routine or complex; new procedures, drugs, instruments)
- Environmental factors (background noise, sound quality, frequent interruptions)

Transcription

- MT knowledge (education, experience, English and medical language fluency, editing skills, familiarity with report types, familiarity with dictating staff)
- MT equipment knowledge (experience on facility's equipment)
- Transcription equipment characteristics (quality, features, maintenance)
- Resource availability (adequate, up-to-date, accessible references; access to other MTs, electronic assistants, and the Internet)
- Environmental factors (ergonomics, distractions)
- Performance expectations (demands for quantity, demands for quality, personnel policies)
- Other responsibilities (answering telephone, filing, etc.)

In addition to transcription responsibilities, many MTs during the past seven years have acquired new responsibilities in the areas of editing and risk management. Some have learned coding, and others are involved with information systems. The historical performance of an individual MT or an entire department can still be determined by establishing the method to quantify productivity and then tracking it over a period of time. If all factors remain the same, productivity will remain the same. However, if one or more dictation or transcription factors change, average productivity (individual and collective) will change. Something as simple as a new chair can alter productivity.

If there are significant differences in productivity, the transcription variables will provide valuable information. If transcriptionist A produces 500 lines a day (a line is anything you want it to be) and transcriptionist B produces 2,000 lines a day, one should explore how to stabilize it.

- Does A need to work on skill-building?
- Does B produce 2,000 lines of quality transcription?
- Does A have responsibilities other than transcription?
- Does A speak the language of medicine as fluently as B?
- Do A and B have equivalent resource materials?
- Does B willingly assist other MTs who have questions?

Equipment failures, lighting, furniture, poor dictating habits, adequate breaks, background noise, or just not feeling well...many factors contribute to variations in an MT's productivity.

The search will likely continue for the average MT. Perhaps he or she will be found lurking behind an average computer screen in an average transcription environment in an average community. Language skills, medical knowledge, and keyboarding coordination will be average, and he or she will receive average dictation from average dictators who perform average procedures on average patients. The difficulty level of the report will be average, and the report will be dictated on average equipment at an average rate and volume in an average dialect. This individual will have access to average resources, and his or her ergonomic surroundings will be average. Management expectations will be average, as will be format design and quality and quantity demands.

d

One thing is certain: There are still more trees in the forest than the woodchuck population can handle in a day, and seven years after our first look at MTs' average production, there is more dictation than all MTs put together can transcribe in a day.

About the author
Pat Forbis, CMT, is CEO of Pat Forbis & Co. She was AAMT's president in 1986 and 1987 and an AAMT staff member from 1990 to 2001.

Appendix E
Full Disclosure in Medical Transcription

Issue

A high priority is placed on fair pay for medical transcriptionists in *A Medical Transcriptionist's Bill of Rights* and in AAMT's strategic plan. This goal is best served when employers and contractors exercise, and employees and clients require, full disclosure of any method used to measure medical transcription productivity.

As used in this paper, the term "contractor" refers to the medical transcription company or the independent medical transcriptionist providing medical transcription services for a "client," which refers to the healthcare facility or medical transcription service for whom the work is done.

AAMT Position

There are numerous ways to measure productivity in medical transcription. The most reliable methods employ quantitative units that are clearly defined, are consistently applied, and are readily verifiable. While favoring no particular method, AAMT strongly urges full disclosure of definitions, formulas, and methods between employer and employee as well as between contractor and client.

In an effort to avoid misunderstandings, to promote a complete, accurate, and timely patient record, and in the interests of ethical business practices, AAMT recommends:

- that quality of patient care documentation is always of primary importance;
- that employers fully disclose to their employees the definitions, methods, and/or formulas used to determine pay, incentives, and benefits;
- that medical transcriptionists determine how they are being paid, and if their pay is based on production, that they verify the measurement of that production;

e

- that contractors explicitly define all units of measure and formulas applied to quantify work done and charges made, and that methods of verification be made available to their clients;
- that clients require full disclosure of the methods and formulas used to measure work done for them and that they verify same, at least on an audit basis.

Production Demands Quality

Medical transcription is not simply the striking of a series of keys to create a string of characters, words, lines, pages, or reports. Rather, it is the process by which raw data in the form of dictation are translated into meaningful communication for the purpose of documenting patient care. This translation and the fund of knowledge behind it demonstrate that quality is always of primary importance in patient care documentation.

Summary

To facilitate the goal of fair pay for medical transcriptionists, and in the interest of ethical business practices, AAMT strongly urges full disclosure of the methods and formulas for determining pay and charges—between employer and employee as well as between contractor and client.

Note: This position paper supersedes any prior AAMT position papers related to productivity measures.

Appendix F
Language Standards

by John H. Dirckx, MD

Q In your column and elsewhere I often see medical terms called "irregular" or "incorrect," including ones that are in constant use and are in all the dictionaries. Who ultimately decides whether a medical term is right or wrong? Are there official committees that rule on these things? Can a correct term become wrong or vice versa?

A A term or expression can be judged right or wrong, apt or unacceptable, regular or deviant according to a variety of standards, the most important of which are listed below.

1. In applying the standard of **usage**, one inquires how widely a language practice is accepted by the community of language users. This is the standard that most modern dictionaries, including medical dictionaries, seek to establish. It is important to recognize, however, that the most diligent lexicographer cannot claim to have sampled more than an infinitesimal fraction of the actual language practices of a population, and that by the time a dictionary has been printed and distributed, its assessments of usage may already be somewhat out of date. Despite these shortcomings, dictionaries and other reference works (glossaries, grammars, style manuals) that purport to record current usage are the most useful and reliable authorities available to writers, editors, and medical transcriptionists.

2. One can also apply an **etymologic** or historical standard, asking how faithfully a word preserves the form and meaning of its earliest known origins. By this standard, a great many of our most-used technical terms, including all of those based on metaphor (*cervix* 'neck', cardiac *chamber*, *muscle* 'little mouse') could be judged aberrant. Persons who assign primary importance to etymologic standards of correctness

the substitute terms are obvious euphemisms, such as *developmentally challenged* for *mentally retarded* and *differently abled* for *disabled*. Others are simply variant terms that have received the blessing, for the time being, of the invisible trend-setters, such as *African American* for *black* and *sexually transmitted disease* for *venereal disease*. Also in this category is gender-neutral language, which requires the speaker or writer to avoid any implication of gender that is not relevant to the subject matter. In gender-neutral language, terms such as *manpower* and *waitress* are replaced with alternatives such as *productiveness* and *server*. The generic masculine pronoun *(he, him, himself, his)* and adjective *(his)* must either yield to a cumbersome formula *(he or she, him or her, himself or herself, his or hers, his or her)* or be expunged through a rephrasing of the material—even to the extent of adopting a colloquial laxness of grammar *(Each patient must form their own judgment and make their own decision accordingly)*.

9. An **esthetic** standard takes into account such abstract qualities of language as poetic imagery, rhythm, and euphony. The application of such standards is highly subjective at best and often becomes a matter of individual taste. Grammarians of the old school based many of their rules, some of which survive today, on such considerations. For example, some still favor the rule that forbids adding the comparative suffix *-er* or the superlative *-est* to adjectives of more than one syllable. According to this rule, *most common* is preferable to *commonest*.

10. There is also a **social** standard, according to which the language practices of educated and cultivated persons are automatically assumed to be correct, and deviations from these practices are condemned as "substandard." But who is entitled to decide for the rest of us what is "refined" or "educated" language? Lexicographers used to assume this authority, but few modern dictionaries contain usage labels based strictly on upper-class speech and writing practices.

11. The **nomenclatures** of certain basic sciences and branches of medicine have been defined within fairly narrow limits by various official or quasi-official boards and associations. The spelling and meaning of

f

terms pertaining to anatomy, histology, embryology, chemistry, pharmacology (both generic names and brand names), and the taxonomy of plants (including pathogenic bacteria and fungi) and animals (including parasites and disease vectors) have been fixed in this way. Some medical specialty boards and government agencies have established official definitions for terms concerning their areas of interest or influence. For example, the *Diagnostic and Statistical Manual of Mental Disorders* published by the American Psychiatric Association contains definitions, in the form of diagnostic criteria, for all currently recognized mental diseases. Although these official nomenclatures are widely accepted and are recorded in technical dictionaries and other reference works, changes in official terminology penetrate very slowly into workaday medical speech and writing. For example, eponymic terms such as *fallopian tube* and *eustachian tube*, which were rejected from anatomic terminology several decades ago, continue in wide use in preference to the official *uterine tube* and *auditory tube*.

12. Institutions and organizations such as hospitals, HMOs, and transcription services often find it expedient to create **style manuals** laying down rules or guidelines on certain aspects of written language, such as abbreviations, capitalization, punctuation, and the use of numerals and units of measure. Such rules may be developed in response to local conditions (such as the rampant proliferation of arbitrary abbreviations in written records or dictation, or an unacceptable diversity in format and styling among transcriptionists) or may even reflect the idiosyncratic preferences of individuals in authority. Hence the standards prescribed may vary considerably from one institution to another. In contrast, *The AAMT Book of Style*, which provides medical transcriptionists with information and guidance on a wide range of issues in medical language as it is used in patients' everyday medical reports, is a consensus document that adopts a broader, more mature, and more rational perspective. Other authoritative reference works on medical language are the *American Medical Association Manual of Style*, published by Lippincott Williams & Wilkins, and *Scientific Style and Format: the CBE Manual for Authors, Editors, and Publishers* issued by the Council of Biology

Editors; these latter two style manuals are specifically intended for authors preparing more formal medical manuscripts for publication.

Finally, because there is a strong subjective element in our experience and perception of language, few of us can resist using our own language practices as the ultimate test of correctness.

Although each of the criteria of aptness or correctness listed above has its own kind of validity, none of them can be applied in an arbitrary or absolute way, much less enforced. Some of these standards overlap others, while, on the other hand, some criteria of correctness are incompatible with other criteria. In judging whether a given language practice is right or wrong, one should evaluate it in the light of relevant circumstances, consult appropriate reference works, decide which standards are applicable, and try to assign each its due weight.

About the author

John H. Dirckx, MD, has been medical director of the Student Health Center at the University of Dayton (Ohio) since 1968. He has written several books and numerous articles on the language, literature, and history of medicine, including textbooks and workbooks for medical transcriptionists. He edited *Stedman's Concise Medical Dictionary for the Health Professions* (Lippincott Williams & Wilkins, 2001). He is also an advisor to the *Journal of the American Association for Medical Transcription (JAAMT)* and authors the "Medical Language" column that has appeared regularly in *JAAMT* since 1984.

Appendix G
Modifying the Patient Record: Corrections, Revisions, Additions, and Addenda

by Harry Rhodes, MBA, RHIA

Work life in health information management would be so much easier if only there were a single national uniform law for corrections, revisions, additions, and addenda. Instead, what exists is a patchwork of laws, standards, guidelines, and best practices. There is not even a unified body of laws to refer to for guidance. The existing state of confusion proves to be very challenging for health information professionals. Questions regarding the appropriate way to process corrections, revisions, additions, and addenda are among the most common types of professional practice questions received at AHIMA. When providing advice on this topic, we find that direction is available from a number of sources.

- The Uniform Rules of Evidence
- The Federal Rules of Evidence 803
- State laws and regulations
- The HIPAA Privacy Final Rule, Section 164.526
- ASTM E31 standards
- HL7 standards

By collectively drawing guidance from each of these sources, a healthcare enterprise can develop a workable policy and procedure.

The Uniform Rules of Evidence
Statements made outside the court and offered as proof of an occurrence are considered hearsay evidence. Normally, hearsay evidence is considered unreliable. Anyone can make a claim that someone consented to, said, or did something at another time and place. The party wishing to have such records accepted as evidence must somehow demonstrate the reliability of the record.

g

The most common type of exception is the business record exception. Under this exception records maintained in the regular course of business are considered admissible as evidence. Medical records fall under the business record exception provided that the method of record keeping conforms to certain established guidelines:

- The record was made in the regular course of business.
- The entries in the record were made at or near the time of the matter recorded.
- The entries were made by the individual within the enterprise with firsthand knowledge of the acts, events, conditions, and opinions.
- Process controls and checks must exist to ensure the reliability and accuracy of the record.
- Policies and procedures must exist to protect the record from alteration and tampering.
- Policies and procedures must exist to prevent loss of stored data.

The Federal Rule of Evidence 803

The Federal Rule of Evidence 803 is very similar to the Uniform Rules of Evidence, except that the federal rule addresses medical records admitted as evidence in federal criminal and civil cases.

Under the Federal Rule of Evidence, a record meets the definition provided

- it is part of the normal course of business to prepare the record in question;
- the record was made at or near the time the act, event, or discussion occurred; and
- the record was prepared by the individual with firsthand knowledge of the events, actions, or opinions.

The rules of evidence and the business record rule provide a strong foundation for the enterprise seeking to develop policies and procedures. In order to ensure the admissibility of the medical record as evidence, the enterprise must first establish policies and procedures that address

- Author authentication
- Medical record access control
- Medical record archiving and retention
- Medical record security
- Medical record disaster recovery policies and procedures

By establishing controls over the creation of medical records, enterprises can ensure the nonrepudiation of corrections, revisions, additions, and addenda made in the normal course of business.

Ultimately, by controlling the how, who, where, and when of creating the medical record, the enterprise establishes the methodology for performing valid corrections, revisions, additions, and addenda.

State Laws and Regulations

Many, but not all, states have laws and regulations that provide guidance on the proper circumstances and methodology for correcting or amending a medical record. State laws and regulations are often quite general and subject to interpretation. Arkansas medical record correction law addresses paper medical records but not electronic. California law states that "altering or modifying the medical record of any person, with fraudulent intent, or creating any false medical record, with fraudulent intent, constitutes unprofessional conduct. In addition to any other disciplinary action, the Division of Medical Quality or the California Board of Podiatric Medicine may impose a civil penalty of five hundred dollars ($500) for violations."[1] However, California law does not provide guidance on the appropriate means of correcting or amending the medical record.

g

Illinois law provides clear guidance on how corrections and supplementation are to be made in the electronic medical record. "The system shall require that corrections or supplementation of previously authenticated entries shall be made by additional entries, separately authenticated and made subsequent in time to the original entry."[2]

HIPAA Privacy Final Rule—Amendment of Protected Health Information

The HIPAA privacy final rule, published on December 28, 2000, provides an individual with the right to have the covered entity amend protected health information or medical records provided that the information is part of the designated record set.

The process outlined in the final rule requires

- that the records affected by the amendment be identified and appended or otherwise linked to the location of the amendment;
- that the covered entity make a reasonable effort to inform individuals impacted by the amendment within a reasonable time, and to provide the amendment within a reasonable time; and
- that a covered entity which is informed by another covered entity of an amendment to the original record amend the protected information in their records.

The HIPAA privacy rule provides a good model for the notification of other healthcare providers that are recipients of health information regarding corrections and amendments to the parent medical record.

ASTM E31 Standards

The ASTM electronic medical record standard *Electronic Authentication of Health Care Information, E1762-95*, Section 8, introduces and defines three types of authentication methods for correcting and amending medical record entries.

1. Addendum Signature: The signature on a new amended document of an individual who has corrected, edited, or amended an original health information document.

2. Modification Signature: The signature on an original document of an individual who has generated a new amended document.

3. Administrative (Error/Edit) Signature: The signature of an individual who is certifying that the document is invalidated by an error(s), or is placed in the wrong chart.

The ASTM model provides a method of tracking amendments and corrections to ensure that only the appropriate individual makes any changes to the medical record.[3]

HL7 Standards

The HL7 standards identify and define the types of errors and corrections that occur in the medical record. For each of the identified errors and corrections HL7 has developed the appropriate computer messages used to communicate the corrections and addenda to disparate computer systems.

HL7 standards provide scenarios for each of the following correction and amendment situations:

1. Creating an addendum: "Author dictates additional information as an addendum to a previously transcribed document. A new document is transcribed. This addendum has its own new unique document ID that is linked to the original document via the parent ID. Addendum document notification is transmitted. This creates a composite document."

2. Correcting errors discovered in a document that has not been made available for patient care: "Errors, which need to be corrected, are discovered in a document. The original document is edited, and an edit notification is sent."

3. Correcting errors discovered in the original document that has been made available for patient care: "Errors discovered in a document are corrected. The original document is replaced with the revised document. The replacement document has its own new unique document ID that

g

is linked to the original document via the parent ID. The availability status of the original document is changed to 'obsolete' but the original document should be retained in the system for historical reference. Document replacement notification is sent."

4. Notification of a canceled document: "When the author dictated a document, the wrong patient identification was given, and the document was transcribed and sent to the wrong patient's record. When the error is discovered, a cancellation notice is sent to remove the document from general access in the wrong patient's record. In these cases, a reason should be supplied in the cancellation message. To protect patient privacy, the correct patient's identifying information should not be placed on the erroneous document that is retained in the wrong patient's record for historical reference. A new document notification and content will be created using the T02 event marker (original document notification and content event) and sent for association with the correct patient's record."

The HL7 standard provides an excellent process for the communication and tracking of medical record addendum and correction.[4]

ASTM E2184, Standard Specification for Healthcare Document Formats

The ASTM committee E31 on Healthcare Informatics has developed a standard specification that addresses requirements for the heading, arrangement, and appearance of sections and subsections when used within an individual's healthcare documents. Within the standard specification, two issues that impact medical record corrections and amendments are addressed and defined: author accountability and record amendments.

Accountability (section 9.22): The document's author or other person responsible for entering into the record the author's statements shall be identified, as well as the date and place of origination and of entry.

Amendments (section 9.24): Amendments to the original document shall be identified by the heading AMENDMENT in all capital letters. Amendments may be corrections or addenda to the original document. Each shall meet the specifications for accountability as specified in 9.22.

This ASTM standard specification clearly establishes the author as the party responsible for all entries into the medical record, including corrections and amendments, and that all amendments to the medical record must be clearly identified.

Summary

Drawing collectively from these laws, standards, guidelines, and best practices, a healthcare enterprise can develop an effective and valid policy and procedure for the correction, revision, addition, and addenda of health information contained within the medical record.

The key characteristics of an effective policy and procedure include

- Author authentication and accountability
- Clear indication of correction or amendment date and time
- Policies and procedures that prevent unauthorized alteration of documents
- Clear delineation of parent document
- Clear delineation of corrected or amended document
- Notification of health information recipients when amendments and corrections occur
- Retention of the parent document for historical reference

Though it is true that no single national law that addresses medical record correction and amendment exists, enough guidance is available to allow healthcare providers to develop a workable policy and procedure to address the creation of valid medical record corrections and amendments.

Footnotes:

1. *The Complete Legal Guide to Healthcare Records Management.* New York, NY: McGraw-Hill, Inc, 2000.

2. Ibid.

3. American Society for Testing and Materials. *2001 Annual Book of ASTM Standards, Vol 14.01. Health Informatics,* West Conshoshocken, PA: 2001.

4. *Health Level Seven, Version 2.4.* Ann Arbor, MI, 2000; available online at www.hl7.org.

Additional References:

- *Comprehensive Guide to Electronic Health Records.* New York, NY: Faulkner & Gray, Inc. 2000.

- Rhodes, Harry. "On the Line: Professional Practice Solutions." *Journal of AHIMA* 69(7): 65-66, 1998.

- "Standards for Privacy of Individually Identifiable Health Information; Final Rule." 45 CFR Part 164. *Federal Register* 65, no. 250 (December 28, 2000); available on-line at http://aspe/hhs.gov/admnsimp/.

About the author:

Harry Rhodes, MBA, RHIA, is Director of HIM Products and Services for the American Health Information Management Association (AHIMA). He serves as a resource to AHIMA members and outside organizations on health information professional practice guidelines through articles, publications, presentations, and consultations.

Appendix H
Soundalikes

abdominal	pertaining to the abdomen
abominable	detestable; unpleasant or disagreeable
abduction	moving away from (often dictated as "a-b-duction")
adduction	drawing toward (often dictated as "a-d-duction")
aberrant	wandering; abnormal
apparent	clear or obvious; visible
abject	existing in a low condition, as in *abject poverty*
object	to oppose (v); something on which one is focused (n)
ablation	surgical removal
oblation	religious offering
accent	characteristic pronunciation
ascent	rising or moving upward; upward slope or incline
assent	to agree with (v); agreement (n)
accept	to receive willingly; to regard as proper
except	other than; to leave out or exclude
access	means of approach; the ability or right to approach
axis	center
excess	more than usual

acetic	sour
acidic	acid-forming
aesthetic	characterized by increased awareness of beauty
ascitic	pertaining to an accumulation of serous fluid in the abdominal cavity
asthenic	pertaining to or characterized by a lack or loss of energy
esthesic	mental perception of sensation
esthetic	improvement in appearance
Acufex	arthroscopic instruments
Acuflex	an intraocular lens
adverse	contrary to one's interests; undesirable, unwanted, as in *adverse reaction*
averse	having a feeling of dislike or revulsion, as in *averse to taking risks*
advice	opinion about what should be done (n)
advise	to counsel, recommend, or inform (v)
aerogenous	gas-producing
erogenous	arousing erotic feelings, as in *erogenous zone*
affect	to influence (v), as in *he affected her deeply*; external expression of emotion (n), as in *a flat affect* (psych)
effect	to bring about (v), as in *effect a change*; result (n), as in *cause and effect*
afferent	toward a center
efferent	outward from a center
affusion	act of pouring a liquid on
effusion	liquid which escapes into tissue
infusion	introduction of a liquid solution through a vein or tissue
alfa	international spelling for alpha, as in interferon alfa
alpha	first letter of the Greek alphabet; the first one; the beginning

The American Association for Medical Transcription

allude	make reference to
elude	evade
elute	extract or remove
allusion	indirect but pointed meaning or reference
elution	separation by washing of one solid from another
illusion	erroneous perception of reality
alkalosis	increased alkalinity of blood and tissues
ankylosis	immobilization of a joint
all	the whole amount
awl	a pointed instrument
alternate	a person acting in the place of another, as in *an alternate delegate* (n); to do by turns (v)
alternating	happening by turns, as in *alternating movements*
alternative	a choice between two possibilities, as in *the only alternative*
AMA	against medical advice, as in *the patient signed out AMA*
ANA	antinuclear antibody
anecdote	an amusing or interesting short story
antidote	a remedy for counteracting a poison
anergia	inactivity
inertia	inability to move spontaneously
anuresis	retention of urine in the bladder
enuresis	involuntary discharge of urine after the age at which control should have been achieved; bed-wetting

h

h

aphagia	refusal or inability to swallow
aphakia	absence of the lens of the eye, most commonly caused by extraction of a cataract
aphasia	speech disorder that involves a defect or loss of the power of expression by speaking, writing, or signing; also inability to comprehend spoken or written language
aplasia	lack of development of an organ or tissue
apposition	placing side by side or next to
opposition	contrary action or condition
assure	to cause to feel sure; to make safe or secure
ensure	to make sure or certain
insure	to make secure; to ensure
astasia	inability to stand due to lack of muscle coordination
ectasia	dilation or expansion
attacks	spells; assaults
Atarax	tranquilizer
ataxia	failure or irregularity of muscle coordination
aura	a sensation or motor phenomenon that precedes a paroxysmal attack such as a seizure
aural	pertaining to the ear
ora	plural of os
oral	pertaining to the mouth
orale	the point in the midline of the maxillary suture that is lingual to the central incisors
avert	to turn aside or turn away
evert	to turn inside out
invert	to turn inside out or upside down; to reverse the order
overt	open to view

BAER	brainstem auditory evoked response
bare	nude
Bayer	brand name for aspirin
bear	to tolerate
ball valve	a heart valve
bivalve	consisting of two similar but separable parts
Beaver	brand name of a series of blades, knives, and keratomes
Deaver	retractor
bolus	a single, rather large mass or quantity of a drug or medication that is administered either orally or intravenously
bullous	relating to bullae
caliber	the diameter of a projectile, usually a bullet; the diameter of a canal or tube
calipers	a compass-like instrument used for measuring thicknesses, such as skinfolds
callous	hard like a callus; hardened in mind or feelings, as in *a callous attitude*
callus	a hardened or thickened area of skin; the meshwork of woven bone that forms at the site of a healing fracture, as in callus formation
carotid	artery
parotid	gland
caudal	a position more toward the tail; often used as a synonym for inferior
coddle	to pamper
Cottle	a manufacturer of surgical instruments
cease	to stop doing; to come to an end
seize	to grab; to take by force; to convulse

h

cecal	pertaining to the cecum
fecal	pertaining to feces
thecal	pertaining to an enclosing case or sheath, as in *thecal sac*
cede	yield or grant, as in the tennis player was forced to cede the point to her opponent
seat	to cause or assist to sit down; to fix firmly in place, as with components of a joint replacement
seed	semen; a small shell used in application of radiation therapy
celiotomy	surgical incision into the abdominal cavity
ciliotomy	surgical division of the ciliary nerves
cell	smallest unit of life capable of existence
cella	an enclosure or compartment
sella	a saddle-shaped depression, as in *sella turcica*
cellular	consisting of cells; porous
sellar	pertaining to the sella turcica
cerise	deep to vivid purplish red
cerous	pertaining to or containing the metallic element cerium
scirrhous	pertaining to or of the nature of a hard cancer
serous	pertaining to or resembling serum
cholic	an acid; relating to bile
colic	acute abdominal pain
chordae	plural of chorda; any cord or sinew
chordee	downward bowing of the penis

cilium	a hairlike projection from a cell
psyllium	the seed of a plant that is used as a mild laxative
circumcise	to remove the foreskin of the penis
circumscribe	to mark off carefully
cirrhosis	liver disease
xerosis	abnormal dryness, as seen in the eyes, skin, or mouth
cite	to quote as an authority or example; to mention as an illustration
-cyte	cell
sight	the function of seeing
site	a place or location
clonus	alternating muscular contraction and relaxation in rapid succession
conus	resembling a cone in shape
cornice	a decorative band
CNS	central nervous system
C&S	culture and sensitivity
collum	the neck
column	a pillar-like structure
complement	that which completes or makes perfect
compliment	an expression of praise or admiration
continence	self-restraint; the ability to retain urine or feces
continents	land masses of the world
continual	recurring frequently
continuous	going on without interruption

h

council	an executive or advisory body
counsel	advice given as a result of a consultation
corollary	something that naturally follows
coronary	pertaining to the heart
creatine	high-energy phosphate
creatinine	product excreted in urine; a diagnostic indicator of kidney function
keratan	a sulfate found in the cornea and in skeletal tissues
keratin	scleroprotein that forms the primary components of epidermis, hair, nails, and horny tissues
cremation	consumption by fire
crenation	abnormal notch found on microscopic exam of an erythrocyte
crus	a term used to designate a leg-like part
crux	a decisive point, as in *crux of the matter*
cytotoxin	a toxin or antibody that has a toxic action on cells of a specific organ
Cytoxan	an antineoplastic drug
sitotoxin	food poisoning
decision	a choice made among options
discission	an incision or cutting into
denervation	loss of nerve supply
enervation	loss of nervous energy
innervation	supply of nerves to a part

dental	relating to teeth or dentistry
dentil	one of a series of small rectangular blocks forming a molding
denticle	a conical pointed projection
identical	the same
desperate	frantic
disparate	markedly distinct in quality
device	equipment or mechanism designed for a purpose
devise	to plan, design, or contrive
diaphysis	the body or shaft of a long bone that ossified from a primary center
diathesis	an inborn tendency to develop certain diseases or other abnormal conditions
diarrhea	abnormally loose and frequent bowel movements
diuria	a crystalline substance derivable from two molecules or urea
diuresis	excretion of abnormally high amounts of urine
discreet	a judicious reserve in one's speech or behavior
discrete	separate or individually distinct, as in *discrete mass*
dissension	strong disagreement; discord
distention	state of being distended or enlarged
dysphagia	difficulty in swallowing
dysphasia	difficulty in speaking
dystaxia	difficulty in controlling voluntary movement
dystectia	defective closure of the neural tube, resulting in malformation
Ebstein	angle; anomaly; disease
Epstein	Epstein-Barr virus, disease

h

eczema	a type of dermatitis
exemia	loss of fluid from blood vessels
ejection	expelling, throwing out
ingestion	taking of food or liquid into the body through the mouth
injection	a shot; congestion
elicit	to bring out, as in *elicit a response*
illicit	illegal, as in *illicit drugs*
emanate	to flow out or proceed from; to originate from
eminence	a prominence or projection, particularly of bone
eminent	important, well known, prominent
imminent	likely or about to occur
enema	injection of fluid into the rectum
intima	innermost structure
intimal	pertaining to the inner layer of a blood vessel
ephedrine	an alkaloid
epinephrine	a catecholamine
Excedrin	a pain reliever for headaches
erasable	removable with an eraser
irascible	easily provoked to anger
ethanal	acetaldehyde
ethinyl	ethynyl
ethanol	alcohol
ethenyl	vinyl
eyes and nose	parts of the anatomy above the lips
I's & O's	intake and output

facial	pertaining to the face
fascial	pertaining to or of the nature of fascia
faucial	pertaining to the passage from the mouth to the pharynx

false	not true
falx	a sickle-shaped organ or structure, as in *falx cerebri*

farther	physical distance, as in *driving farther than planned*
further	extension of time or degree, as in *further care before discharge*

fascicle	a band or bundle of fibers, as in muscle or nerve
vesical	pertaining to the bladder
vesicle	a small sac containing fluid, as in *the lesions seen in chickenpox*

faze	to cause to be disconcerted, as in *the problem didn't faze him*
phase	a stage of development
phrase	a group of words

fibers	slender structures or filaments
fibrose	to form fibrous tissue
fibrous	composed of or containing fibers

filamentous	composed of long threadlike structures
velamentous	in the form of a sheet or veil

filiform	thread-shaped; a slender bougie
phalliform	shaped like a penis
piliform	shaped like or resembling hair

flanges	projecting borders or edges
phalanges	plural of phalanx; bones of the fingers or toes

h

fornix	arch-shaped roof of an anatomical space
pharynx	the throat (often mispronounced as "fair-nix")
fovea	a cup-shaped pit or depression
folia	plural of folium, a leaf-like structure
phobia	a fear or morbid dread
gaited	walking or running in a certain manner, as in *a gaited horse*
gated	an entrance or opening, as in *gated magnetic resonance cardiac imaging*
glands	cells that function as secretory or excretory organs
glans	a conical-shaped structure, as in *glans penis*
Gleason	score for grading prostate carcinoma
Glisson	capsule; tissue covering the liver
glisten	to sparkle
glucoside	a glycoside in which the sugar content is glucose
glycoside	any of the class of compounds that yield a sugar and an aglycon upon hydrolysis, as in *cardiac glycoside*
graft	tissue implanted from one point to another
graph	a diagram with connecting points
hear	to listen
here	where you are right now
hemolysis	disruption of the integrity of the erythrocyte membrane causing release of hemoglobin
homolysis	lysis of a cell by extracts of the same type of tissue
Hertel	rigid dilator stone forceps; exophthalmometer
Hurthle	as in *Hurthle cell adenoma, Hurthle cell carcinoma, Hurthle cell tumor*

heterotopia	displacement of parts or organs; presence of tissue in an abnormal location
heterotrophia	nutritional disorder
heterotropia	strabismus
holder	a container; a device for immobilizing a part of the body, as in *head holder*
Holter	a heart monitor
HNP	herniated nucleus pulposus
H&P	history and physical
humerus	long bone in upper arm
humorous	funny
ileac	pertaining to the distal portion of the colon
iliac	pertaining to the superior portion of the hip bone
ileum	distal portion of the colon
ilium	superior portion of the hip bone
inanimate	without life or spirit, as in *an inanimate object*
innominate	nameless, as in *an innominate artery*
inanition	loss of vitality
inattention	failure to pay attention
inhibition	self-restriction of freedom of activity
incidence	rate or frequency of occurrence
incidents	single occurrences, events, or happenings
instance	case or example

h

incision	a wound made in surgery
schism	disunion or discord
scission	cleavage; splitting
infarction	necrosis caused by obstruction, as in *myocardial infarction*
infection	invasion of the body by organisms that can cause disease
inflection	change in vocal pitch or loudness; bending forward
infraction	incomplete fracture; breaking of a rule
installation	placing in a position or office
instillation	injecting slowly
irradiate	to treat with radioactivity
radiate	to spread out from a center, as in *the pain radiates into the lower leg*
jewel	a precious stone
joule	a unit of energy
jowl	a fold of flesh hanging from the jaw
karyon	nucleus
kerion	a secondarily infected granulomatous lesion
keloid	a hyperplastic scar
keroid	resembling horn or corneal tissue
kempt	referring to a neat appearance
kept	past tense of keep
labial	pertaining to a lip or lip-like structure
labile	unstable, as in labile blood pressure
lassitude	listlessness
latitude	freedom of choice; plane of reference

leak	an accidental opening that permits substance or information to escape
LEEP	loop electrosurgical procedure (gyn)
LLETZ	laparoscopic laser excision of the transformation zone (gyn)
Leiden	genetic mutation associated with clotting factor V
Leyden	genetic mutation associated with clotting factor IX
lesser	smaller when comparing two things, as in *lesser evil*
lessor	one who conveys property by a lease
liable	responsible for
libel	defamation by written or printed words
libido	sexual desire
livedo	bluish discoloration of skin
lice	parasites
lyse	to break up or disintegrate, as in *lysis of adhesions*
lightening	decreasing in weight
lighting	illumination
lightning	a flash of light produced by electricity in the atmosphere, as in *thunder and lightning*
liver	large gland in the abdomen
livor	discoloration appearing on the body after death
loop	an oval or circular ring formed by bending a vessel or cylindrical organ
loupe	a magnifying glass
loose	not securely attached
lose	to misplace

h

h

mammoplasty	plastic surgery of the breast; mammaplasty
manoplasty	plastic surgery of the hand
meiosis	method of cell division
miosis	contraction of the pupil of the eye
mitosis	method of indirect cell division
mycosis	presence of parasitic fungi in the body
myiasis	infection due to invasion of body tissues or cavities by larvae of dipterous insects
meiotic	pertaining to special cell division
miotic	causing contraction of the pupil of the eye
mitotic	pertaining to indirect division of a cell
myopic	nearsighted
menorrhagia	excessive uterine bleeding
menorrhalgia	painful menstruation; dysmenorrhea
metrorrhagia	uterine bleeding of abnormal amount, occurring at abnormal times
mnemonic	something intended to assist memory
pneumonic	related to or affecting the lungs
modeling	learning by observation and imitation
mottling	a condition of spotting with patches of color
mucous	adjective form of mucus; pertaining to or resembling mucus
mucus	free slime of the mucous membranes
myoclonic	demonstrating one of a series of shock-like muscular contractions, as in *a seizure*
myotonic	exhibiting delayed relaxation of a muscle after a strong contraction, or prolonged contraction after mechanical stimulation

nucleide	a compound of nucleic acid with a metallic element
nuclide	a species of atom
osteal	bony
ostial	pertaining to an ostium
pain	discomfort, distress, or agony
pane	a segment of window glass
pair	two of something
pare	to trim or remove skin
palate	roof of the mouth
palette	an oval board with a thumb-hole used by artists to mix their paints
pallet	a portable platform; a temporary bed made of folded blankets
palpable	may be felt with the hand
palpebral	pertaining to the eyelid
palpation	feeling with the fingers
palpitation	an abnormal, rapid heartbeat
papillation	a covering of small round protuberances
parotic	near the ear
perotic	characterized by perosis
porotic	favoring growth of connective tissue
peal	to ring, as a bell
peel	to strip away a layer
perfusion	the act of pouring over or through
profusion	abundance
protrusion	a jutting-out from the surrounding surface

h

perineal	pertaining to the perineum
peritoneal	pertaining to the peritoneum
peroneal	pertaining to the outer or fibular side of the leg
perspective	one's ideas; a way of looking at something
prospective	in the future, potential
phenol	carbolic acid
phenyl	derived from benzene
pheresis	removal from a donor; separation and retransfusion
-phoresis	word ending indicating transmission
plain	not fancy; radiograph, as in *plain abdomen*
plane	anatomic level, as in *the sagittal plane*
pleuritis	inflammation of the pleura
pruritus	itching
pleural	pertaining to the pleura of the lung
plural	more than one
precede	to go before
proceed	to continue on
precedent	coming before; an example
president	a governmental leader
prescribe	to order; to advise
proscribe	to banish or denounce; to forbid

principal	a leader, as in *high school principal*; a main participant, as in *principal diagnosis*; the main body of an estate or financial holding
principle	a basic truth; a rule or standard
Procan	SR; an antiarrhythmic medication
procaine	a local anesthetic
prostate	a gland of the male urinary tract
prostrate	stretched out with the face upon the ground
rostrate	having a beak-like structure
prostatic	relating to the prostate gland
prosthetic	pertaining to an artificial device that replaces a body part
psoriasis	a dermatosis
siriasis	sunstroke
psychosis	mental disorder
sycosis	pustular inflammation of hair follicles
quiet	without noise
quite	completely
radical	extreme, drastic, or innovative; elements or atoms in an uncombined state, as in free radicals
radicle	smallest branch of a vessel
rectus	straight structure
rhexis	rupture of an organ
rictus	fissure or cleft; a gaping expression
ructus	a belching of wind

h

refection	recovery
reflection	bending back
refraction	deviation of light
regard	to look at or observe; to relate or refer to
regards	good wishes
regime	a form of government
regimen	a system of treatment, medication, or diet designed to achieve certain ends
role	the part one plays
roll	to turn over (v); a list for attendance purposes (n)
saccadic	simultaneous movements of both eyes that are involuntary in changing the point of fixation
psychotic	pertaining to a severe mental disorder
scatoma	a tumor-like mass in the rectum
scotoma	an area of depressed vision in the visual field
scleredema	unusual swelling of the facial area
scleroderma	chronic thickening and hardening of the skin
xeroderma	a mild form of ichthyosis
serial	arranged in a series
sural	pertaining to the calf of the leg
shoddy	of poor workmanship or quality
shotty	resembling buckshot, as in *shotty nodes*
statue	a three-dimensional work of art
statute	a law enacted by a legislative body

subtle	so slight as to be difficult to detect or analyze
supple	moving or bending with agility; limber
vary	to change
very	extreme; a high degree
venous	relating to a vein
Venus	second planet from the sun; the Roman goddess of love
vial	a small bottle
vile	despicable or abhorrent

h

Appendix I
Professional Credentials and Academic Degrees

See the following topics for guidance on capitalization:
credentials, professional
degrees, academic
fellow, Fellow

BS	Bachelor of Science
BSN	Bachelor of Science in Nursing
CM	Certified Midwife
CMT	Certified Massage Therapist
CMT	Certified Medical Transcriptionist
CNM	Certified Nurse Midwife
CNMT	Certified Nuclear Medicine Technologist
CO	Certified Orthoptist
COMT	Certified Ophthalmic Medical Technologist
CPFT	Certified Pulmonary Function Technologist
CPNP	Certified Pediatric Nurse Practitioner
CRT	Certified Respiratory Therapist
CVT	Certified Veterinary Technician
DC	Doctor of Chiropractic
DDS	Doctor of Dental Surgery
DMD	Doctor of Dental Medicine
DO	Doctor of Osteopathy
DPM	Doctor of Podiatric Medicine
DVM	Doctor of Veterinary Medicine
EdD	Doctor of Education
EMT	Emergency Medical Technician
EMT-P	Emergency Medical Technician-Paramedic
FAAFP	Fellow of the American Academy of Family Physicians
FACCP	Fellow of the American College of Chest Physicians

FACEP	Fellow of the American College of Emergency Physicians
FACNM	Fellow of the American College of Nurse-Midwives
FACP	Fellow of the American College of Physicians
FACR	Fellow of the American College of Radiology
FACR	Fellow of the American College of Rheumatology
FACS	Fellow of the American College of Surgeons
FNP	Family Nurse Practitioner
FRCP	Fellow of the Royal College of Physicians
GNP	Geriatric Nurse Practitioner
JD	Doctor of Jurisprudence
LPN	Licensed Practical Nurse
LVN	Licensed Vocational Nurse
LVT	Licensed Veterinary Technician
MA	Master of Arts
MBA	Master of Business Administration
MD	Doctor of Medicine
ME	Medical Examiner
MEd	Master of Education
MFA	Master of Fine Arts
MHA	Master of Hospital Administration
MN	Master of Nursing
MPA	Master of Public Administration
MPH	Master of Public Health
MS	Master of Science
MSN	Master of Science in Nursing
MSPH	Master of Science in Public Health
MSW	Master of Social Work; Master of Social Welfare
MT	Medical Technologist
MT(ASCP)	Registered Medical Technologist (American Society of Clinical Pathologists)
MTA	Medical Technical Assistant
ND	Doctor of Naturopathic Medicine
NP	Nurse Practitioner
OD	Doctor of Optometry

OT	Occupational Therapist
OTR	Occupational Therapist, Registered
OTR/L	Occupational Therapist, Registered (and licensed by state)
PA	Physician Assistant
PA-C	Physician Assistant-Certified
PharmD	Doctor of Pharmacy
PhD	Doctor of Philosophy
PNP	Pediatric Nurse Practitioner
PsyD	Doctor of Psychology
PT	Physical Therapist
RCS	Registered Cardiac Sonographer
RD	Registered Dietitian
RDCS	Registered Diagnostic Cardiac Sonographer
RDMS	Registered Diagnostic Medical Sonographer
RHIA	Registered Health Information Administrator
RHIT	Registered Health Information Technologist
RN	Registered Nurse
RNC	Registered Nurse Certified
ROUB	Registered Ophthalmic Ultrasound Biometrist
RPFT	Registered Pulmonary Function Therapist
RRT	Registered Respiratory Therapist
RVT	Registered Vascular Technologist
RVT	Registered Veterinary Technician

Appendix J
American Cities and States

Abbreviation standard	USPS	State	Cities
Ala.	AL	Alabama	Birmingham† Mobile Montgomery*
	AK	Alaska	Anchorage† Fairbanks Juneau*
Ariz.	AZ	Arizona	Phoenix* Tucson
Ark.	AR	Arkansas	Fort Smith Little Rock*
Calif.	CA	California	Los Angeles† Sacramento* San Diego San Francisco San Jose
Colo.	CO	Colorado	Colorado Springs Denver*
Conn.	CT	Connecticut	Bridgeport† Hartford* New Haven
Del.	DE	Delaware	Dover* Wilmington†
Fla.	FL	Florida	Jacksonville† Miami Orlando Tallahassee* Tampa
Ga.	GA	Georgia	Atlanta* Augusta
	HI	Hawaii	Hilo Honolulu*

According to the US Census Bureau's 2000 report

* = capital

† = largest city (if the capital isn't)

Abbreviation		State	Cities
standard	USPS		
Ida.	ID	Idaho	Boise* Pocatello
Ill.	IL	Illinois	Chicago† Springfield*
Ind.	IN	Indiana	Ft. Wayne Indianapolis* South Bend
Ia.	IA	Iowa	Cedar Rapids Des Moines* Sioux City
Kan.	KS	Kansas	Kansas City Topeka* Wichita†
Ken.	KY	Kentucky	Frankfort* Lexington† Louisville
La.	LA	Louisiana	Baton Rouge* New Orleans† Shreveport
Me.	ME	Maine	Augusta* Bangor Portland†
Md.	MD	Maryland	Annapolis* Baltimore†
Mass.	MA	Massachusetts	Boston* Springfield Worchester
Mich.	MI	Michigan	Detroit† Flint Grand Rapids Lansing*
Minn.	MN	Minnesota	Minneapolis† Rochester St. Paul*

According to the US Census
Bureau's 2000 report

* = capital

† = largest city (if the capital isn't)

j

Abbreviation		State	Cities
standard	USPS		
Miss.	MS	Mississippi	Biloxi Gulfport Jackson*
Mo.	MO	Missouri	Jefferson City* Kansas City† St. Louis
Mont.	MT	Montana	Billings† Great Falls Helena*
Neb.	NE	Nebraska	Bellevue Lincoln* Omaha†
Nev.	NV	Nevada	Carson City* Las Vegas† Reno
N.H.	NH	New Hampshire	Concord* Manchester†
N.J.	NJ	New Jersey	Atlantic City Jersey City Newark*
N.M.	NM	New Mexico	Albuquerque† Las Cruces Santa Fe*
N.Y.	NY	New York	Albany* Buffalo New York City† Rochester
N.C.	NC	North Carolina	Charlotte† Raleigh* Winston-Salem
N.D.	ND	North Dakota	Bismarck* Fargo† Grand Forks

According to the US Census Bureau's 2000 report

* = capital

† = largest city (if the capital isn't)

Abbreviation standard	USPS	State	Cities
O.	OH	Ohio	Cincinnati Cleveland Columbus*
Okla.	OK	Oklahoma	Oklahoma City* Tulsa
Ore.	OR	Oregon	Eugene Portland† Salem*
Penn.	PA	Pennsylvania	Harrisburg* Philadelphia† Pittsburgh
R.I.	RI	Rhode Island	Providence* Warwick
S.C.	SC	South Carolina	Charleston Columbia* Greenville
S.D.	SD	South Dakota	Pierre* Rapid City Sioux Falls†
Tenn.	TN	Tennessee	Knoxville Memphis† Nashville*
Tex.	T	Texas	Austin* Dallas Houston† San Antonio
	UT	Utah	Provo Salt Lake City*
Vt.	VT	Vermont	Burlington† Montpelier*
Va.	VA	Virginia	Norfolk Richmond* Virginia Beach†

According to the US Census Bureau's 2000 report

* = capital

† = largest city (if the capital isn't)

j

Abbreviation standard	USPS	State	Cities
Wash.	WA	Washington	Olympia* Seattle† Spokane
W. Va.	WV	West Virginia	Charleston* Huntington Parkersburg
Wis.	WI	Wisconsin	Green Bay Madison* Milwaukee†
Wy.	WY	Wyoming	Casper Cheyenne*
D.C.	DC	District of Columbia	Washington

j

According to the US Census Bureau's 2000 report

* = capital

† = largest city (if the capital isn't)

Bibliography

It is impossible to list all the references used in creating this style manual. The following are those books or other references that were either used extensively or quoted directly.

The AMA Manual of Style, 9th ed. Baltimore: Lippincott Williams & Wilkins, 1998.

The American Heritage Dictionary of the English Language, 4th ed. New York: Houghton Mifflin, 2000.

Blauvelt C. and Nelson F. *Manual of Orthopedic Terminology,* 6th ed. St. Louis: Mosby, 1998.

The Chicago Manual of Style, 14th ed. Chicago: University of Chicago Press, 1993.

Diagnostic and Statistical Manual, 4th edition, text revision (DSM IV-TR). Washington DC: American Psychiatric Association, 2000.

Dorland's Illustrated Medical Dictionary, 29th ed. Philadelphia: W.B. Saunders Company, 2000.

Maggio R. *Talking About People: A Guide to Fair and Accurate Language.* Phoenix, AZ: Oryx Press, 1997.

Stedman's Medical Dictionary, 28th ed. Baltimore: Lippincott Williams & Wilkins, 2000.

Vera Pyle's Current Medical Terminology, 8th ed. Modesto: Heath Professions Institute, 2000.

About AAMT

The American Association for Medical Transcription (AAMT) is a not-for-profit national association for professional medical transcriptionists. AAMT's ongoing mission is to represent and advance the profession of medical transcription and its practitioners.

AAMT offers a variety of membership categories making it possible for both individuals and businesses to contribute to the profession. These membership categories include Practitioner (the medical transcriptionist), Student, Postgraduate, Associate, Corporate, Institutional, Sustaining, and Honorary. Member benefits include the award-winning bimonthly *Journal of the American Association for Medical Transcription (JAAMT)*; discounts on AAMT meetings and conferences, educational and specialty products; toll-free access to AAMT's professional customer service and Help Desk; and networking opportunities both nationally and through nearly 130 local chapters and state/regional associations throughout the United States.

AAMT also administers the Medical Transcriptionist Certification Commission (MTCC) at AAMT, which awards the CMT (certified medical transcriptionist) professional designation.

For more information on the American Association for Medical Transcription and its programs, products, and services, contact:

AAMT
100 Sycamore Avenue
Modesto, CA 95354
(800) 982-2182
Fax: (209) 527-9633
Email: aamt@aamt.org
Website: http://www.aamt.org

Index

Note: Page numbers in boldface refer to the alphabetic (main) entries.

Index

African American, **15**
age referents, **16–18**
ages, **17–18**
ages, using fractions, 181
a.k.a., **18**
alfa, **19**, 490
alkalosis, 491
all, 491
allergies, **19**
allude, 491
allusion, 491
alpha, 490
alphanumeric terms, **20**
alternate, 491
alternate, alternative, **20–21**
alternating, 491
alternative, 491
alternative forms, **21**
although, though, **21–22**
a.m., AM, **22**
AMA (against medical advice), 491
AMA Manual of Style, 162, 217, 221, 267, 279, 289
amino acids, genetics, 188
amount of, **22–23**, 276
ampersand, **23**, 46
ANA (antinuclear antibody), 491
anatomic terms, **24–25**
and, 23
and others, **25**, 237–38
and so forth, **26**, 237–38
and/or, **25**
anecdote, 491
anergia, 491
angles, **26**, 294
ankylosis, 491
antecedents and pronouns, 336
antidote, 491
antigenic specificities, HLA, 207
antigens, 206–07, 246
anuresis, 491

APGAR, **27**
aphagia, 492
aphakia, 492
aphasia, 492
aplasia, 492
apostrophes, **27–28**, 125
apothecary system, 148
apparent, 489
appendages, 13
apposition, 492
appositives, **29–30**, 88
appropriate references, 349
arabic numerals, 279–80, 307
arabic v roman numerals, 279
area, 218
arms, of chromosomes, 185
army, Army, **31**
articles, 1, **31**, 389
as, **32**
as if, as though, **32**
as well as, **32–33**
ascent, 489
ascitic, 490
assent, 489
assistant, associate, **33**
associate, 33
assure, 492
assure, ensure, insure, **34**
astasia, 492
Aster-Coller, 50
asthenic, 490
ASTM, 19, 104, 120, 203, 341, 484–87
Atarax, 492
ataxia, 492
attacks, 492
audit trails, **34**
aura, 492
aural, 492
author, 294
autopsy report, **34**, 454–56
average of, **34**

Index

cremation, 496
crenation, 496
crepitance, creptation, creptus, **115**
Crowe classification, 295
crus, 496
crux, 496
C-section, 290–91
currencies, international, 144–45
-cyte, 495
cytology, 51, 452
cytotoxin, 496
Cytoxan, 496

D

D (dictated), **117**
dangerous abbreviations and dose designations, 461–64
dangling modifiers, **117–18**
dashes, **118–19**, 211
data, datum, **119**
date and time stamp, 178
date dictated, date transcribed, **119–20**, 178
dates, **120–22**
 commas, 89
 virgules, 416
days of the week, **122–23**
Deaver, 493
decade references, in ages, 18
decades, 431–32
deci-, **123**
deciliter (dL), 141
decimal outlines, 301
decimals, decimal units, **123–25**, 218–19
decision, 496
decubitus ulcers, 74
definite article, 31, 389
degrees
 academic, **125–28**, 511–13
 angles, 26
 burns, 72–73
 symbols, **124**, 387
 temperature, 386–87
deka-, **128**

denervation, 496
dental, 497
denticle, 497
dentil, 497
deoxyribonucleic acid (DNA), 141, 187
dependent clause, 80
dependent nonessential clauses, 81–82
depth, **129**
derived names, 313
desperate, 497
device, 497
devise, 497
diabetes mellitus, **129–32**, 130–31
diacritics, 11
diagnosis, **132–35**
 code, 85
 differential, 319
Diagnostic and Statistical Manual of Mental Disorders, 134
diagonal, 415–18
diaphysis, 497
diarrhea, 497
diathesis, 497
dictated but not read, **135–36**
dictated (D), 117
dictation, date of, 119–20
dictation problems, **136–37**, 155–57
dictator, **137**, 294
die of, die from, **138**
differ, different, **138**
differential blood count, 39
differential diagnosis, 135, 319
dilation, dilatation, **138**
dimensions, using fractions, 181
dimensions, using x, 427
Dirckx, John H., MD, 475–80
directional terms, anatomy, 24
dis-, dys-, **138–39**
discharge summary, **139**, 445–46
discission, 496
discreet, 497
discrete, 497

Index

Index

Index

ARAbic